中华传统经典养生术
（汉英对照）

(Chinese- English) Traditional and Classical Chinese Health Cultivation

Chief Producer Li Jie	总策划　李　洁
Chief Compilers Li Jie Xu Feng Xiao Bin Zhao Xiaoting	总主编　李　洁　许　峰　肖　斌　赵晓霆
Chief Translator Han Chouping	总主译　韩丑萍
English Language Reviewer Charles Savona Ventura	英译主审　查尔斯·萨沃纳·文图拉

行步功

U0250683

Xing Bu Gong (Qigong Exercise in Walking)

编著　肖　斌
Compiler　Xiao Bin

翻译　潘　霖
Translator　Pan Lin

上海科学技术出版社
Shanghai Scientific & Technical Publishers

图书在版编目（ＣＩＰ）数据

行步功：汉英对照 / 肖斌编著；潘霖翻译. -- 上
海：上海科学技术出版社，2023.1
（中华传统经典养生术）
ISBN 978-7-5478-6032-8

Ⅰ．①行… Ⅱ．①肖… ②潘… Ⅲ．①气功－健身运
动－基本知识－汉、英 Ⅳ．①R214

中国版本图书馆CIP数据核字（2022）第239928号

Xing Bu Gong（Qigong Exercise in Walking） · 行步功

行步功

编著 肖 斌

上海世纪出版（集团）有限公司
上海 科 学 技 术 出 版 社 出版、发行
（上海市闵行区号景路159弄A座9F-10F）
邮政编码201101 www.sstp.cn
上海当纳利印刷有限公司印刷
开本 787×1092 1/16 印张 10.5
字数 130千字
2023年1月第1版 2023年1月第1次印刷
ISBN 978-7-5478-6032-8 / R·2680
定价：100.00元

内容提要

Summary

行走是人类本能的基本生命活动状态之一，如果能利用行走来练功，将更加方便易行，更有利于传播推广并取得成效。行步功是气功中众多功法中的一部分，分散在各门各派流传的功法之中，主要分为养生健身和习练功夫两大类。我们从众多功法中按儒、释、道、医、武五大类各选一种功法，汇编成本书。

本书所选功法之中，"矮步行功"为古时候儒家与普通大众所习练的功法，简单易行，分为高、中、低三种姿势，其中高、中位适合祛病、养生、健身；中、低位适合练习功夫。"逍遥行步功"为道家所传行步功，通过把肢体导引、站桩桩功和静心冥想相结合，使三调合一，进入一种恍惚杳冥的深层练功态，日久功深，体内真气充足，并起到养生健身、调理脏腑、祛病康复的功用。"佛家行禅法"来自佛家修炼，特别讲究身心相合，通过行走的方式入静入定，长久习练可以进入深层的练功状态。"郭林新气功"总结继承了古代气功导引，三调结合，以行步功的形式防治多种疾病。"八卦行步功"出自功夫门派八卦门，分为八卦行步功（直线蹚泥步）和八卦转掌（走圈蹚泥步）两种，习练日久可以祛病、健身、养生，甚至练出真正的功夫。通过对行步功的研究与习练，希望本书能更好地为人类健康事业服务，为太极健康事业添砖加瓦。

Walking is one of the human beings' instinctive life activities. If walking can be developed as an exercise method to strengthen our bodies, such training will be willingly and widely accepted for its convenience and feasibility. Qigong exercise in walking, a type of qigong, can be found in common qigong exercises. Based on its function, qigong exercise in walking is classified into martial arts exercise and health cultivation exercise. In this book, we selected one exercise from each of the five qigong categories: Confucianism, Buddhism, Taoism, medicine and martial arts.

Among all the exercises, Bent-Leg qigong exercise in walking is practiced by ancient Confucians and ordinary people. This exercise can be classified into three postures: high-position walking, middle-position walking and low-position walking. The practice of high-position walking and middle-position walking can help to achieve wellness and longevity, while low-position walking is suitable for practicing martial arts. Xiao Yao (free and easy) qigong exercise in walking is developed by Taoists. It aims to strengthen the body, supplement the genuine qi and tranquilize the mind through Daoyin, post standing exercise and meditation, eventually achieving the unity of the three regulations to cultivate health. Originating from Buddhists' exercise, walking meditation emphasizes integrating one's body and mind. Long-term practice through walking can make one enter into concentrated meditation. Guo Lin qigong summarizes and carries the legacy of ancient qigong, Daoyin and unity of the three regulations, thus preventing diseases through walking. Ba Gua (Eight-Diagram) qigong exercise in walking originated from Ba Gua martial school. It can be classified into Ba Gua qigong exercise in walking (straight mud-wading walking) and Ba Gua Palm Turning Exercise (circular mud-wading walking). With long-term practice, one can develop real kung fu. By studying, practicing and teaching qigong exercise in walking, I sincerely hope this book can make contributions to health cultivation and Taiji Health.

顾问委员会

Advisory Committee Members

主任

徐建光　陈凯先　严世芸　胡鸿毅

Directors

Xu Jianguang　Chen Kaixian　Yan Shiyun　Hu Hongyi

副主任

王拥军　舒　静　郑林赟　林　勋

Vice Directors

Wang Yongjun　Shu Jing　Zheng Linyun　Lin Xun

学术顾问

林中鹏　林　欣　俞尔科　潘华信　潘华敏
姚玮莉　王　彤　王庆华　刘　华　聂爱国

Academic Advisers

Lin Zhongpeng	Lin Xin	Yu Erke	Pan Huaxin
Pan Huamin	Yao Weili	Wang Tong	Wang Qinghua
Liu Hua	Nie Aiguo		

编纂委员会

Compilation Committee Members

总策划

李 洁

Chief Producer

Li Jie

总主编

李 洁 许 峰 肖 斌 赵晓霆

Chief Compilers

Li Jie Xu Feng Xiao Bin Zhao Xiaoting

副总主编

沈晓东 孙 磊 陆 颖

Vice Chief Compilers

Shen Xiaodong Sun Lei Lu Ying

总主译

韩丑萍

Chief Translator

Han Chouping

副主译

翁 玮 张凯维 潘 霖

Vice Chief Translators

Weng Wei Zhang Kaiwei Pan Lin

项目资助

Acknowledgements

·上海市进一步加快中医药传承创新发展三年行动计划（2021—2023年）"中医药健康素养提升工程"［项目编号：ZY（2021–2023）–0105］

·健康上海行动专项项目（2022—2024年）"名家推广中医传统功法，冠军带动全民健身活动"［项目编号：JKSHZX–2022–04］

· The Three-Year Action Plan for Inheritance, Innovation and Development of Traditional Chinese Medicine in Shanghai (2021–2023) on Improvement of Traditional Chinese Medicine Health Literacy under grant No. ZY(2021–2023)–0105

· Healthy Shanghai Action Project (2022–2024) on Masters Promoting Traditional Chinese Medicine Exercises and Champions Leading Public Fitness Activities under grant No. JKSHZX–2022–04

序

中华传统养生术源远流长，在数千年的发展演化过程中，汲取儒、道、释等与人的生命活动和治病养生有关的文化营养，形成了独特的理论体系和身心锻炼技法。有些技术和方法甚至在砭、针、灸、药之前，是中华民族最早修身养性、祛病延年的重要组成部分。

出土文献马王堆《导引图》、张家山《引书》、战国《行气玉佩铭》等为中华导引术提供了珍贵的考古史料，存世文献《庄子》《吕氏春秋》《黄帝内经》等也有相关理论和方法的记载。此后，导引学术思想不断丰富、发展和创新，20世纪50年代又以"气功"之名呈现于世，闻名海内外。

中华传统导引术和中医养生学是中华民族健康维护的原点，蕴含了中华文明的生生之理。"天人合一"的整体观和辨证观是中华文明的精髓和核心。《道德经》曰：人法地，地法天，天法道，道法自然。整体观既是中国传统哲学的基石，也是中医学和养生学的重要理论基础。中医学认为人体是一个有机的整体，脏腑、经络、精气神等都是有机整体，同时人与社会和自然也是一个整体，相互融合不可分割。

上海市气功研究所在建所三十年之际，提出构建现代气功"气以臻道"学术思想，得到学界广泛响应。研究所总结多年来教学培训经验，汇集成第一批凡八种养生术——易筋经、古音六字诀、逍遥功、八段锦、天柱导引功、松柔功、六合功和放松功，以汉英对照方式出版发行，得到国内外同道的青睐和赞誉。

世界卫生组织（WHO）提出健康新概念："健康不仅为疾病或羸弱之消除，而系体格、精神与社会之完全健康状态。"随着当代世界面临的传染病、慢性疾病、老龄化和精神卫生等健康问题的前所未有的挑战，WHO提出要寻找低成本干预措施，延缓发展态势，减轻经济负担。WHO提出的战略目标之一，就是通过把传统和补充医学服务纳入卫生保健服务供给和自我卫生保健之中，来促进全民健康覆盖。

2016年在WHO指导下,上海中医药大学、上海市中医药研究院成立太极健康中心。该中心秉承以中华传统文化"太极"为标志,以WHO倡导的生理、心理健康及良好社会适应性的健康新理念为目标,以传统中医养生、保健、导引、按蹻、食疗、药膳、心理为技术手段,结合中华太极文化深厚底蕴,整体构建"太极健康"的自我疗愈模式,并推广于世界各地各民族中。李洁教授及其同仁在第一批"中华传统经典养生术"基础上,精选传统导引术以及与日常生活密切相关的站、行、坐、卧方式,汇集第二批凡五种养生术——诸病源候论导引术、站桩功、行步功、卧功、神气五行操等,再次以汉英对照形式出版发行。

我深信这套丛书的出版会对传承中华传统文化,发挥中医药整体观和治未病特色、提升全民中医药健康素养起到良好的促进作用。我深切期待着他们能够再接再厉,不断创新,让中华优秀文化和传统养生术惠及世界各地更多民众。

胡鸿毅

2022年8月

Traditional Chinese health preservation has a long-standing history. Its well-established theoretical system has evolved over thousands of years by integrating Confucianism, Taoism, Buddhism and cultural understanding on human health and disease. As an essential part in promoting health and longevity, some practice methods were long before the emergence of *Bian*-stone, acupuncture, moxibustion and Chinese herbs.

These ancient practice methods have been proved by unearth books including the *Dao Yin Tu* (Daoyin Diagram) in Mawangdui, *Yin Shu* (Book on Daoyin) in Zhangjiashan and *Xing Qi Yu Pei Ming* (Jade Inscriptions on Qi Cultivation) from the Warring States Period, along with the later books such as *Zhuang Zi* (Zhuangzi), *Lü Shi Chun Qiu* (Spring and Autumn of Master Lü), and *Huang Di Nei Jing* (Yellow Emperor's Internal Classic). The academic idea on Daoyin has been further enriched and developed. In 1950s, the Daoyin became known as Qigong.

Traditional Chinese Daoyin and health preservation are essential to the health and wellness of Chinese people and contain the philosophical wisdom of Chinese civilization, which highlights the holistic and dialectic view on man-nature unity. The *Daodejing* states, "Men emulate earth; earth emulates heaven; heaven emulates the Dao; and the Dao emulates spontaneity." The holistic view is both the corner stone of traditional Chinese philosophy and theoretical foundation of Chinese medicine and health preservation. Chinese medicine believes that the human body is an organic whole, including the zang-fu organs, meridians, essence, qi and spirit. In addition, man is inseparable to society and nature.

On the occasion of celebrating the 30th anniversary, Shanghai Qigong Research Institute put forward the academic idea of "Qi-Dao harmony" and compiled a set of eight books (in Chinese and English) on health preservation exercise—*Yi Jin Jing* (Sinew-Transformation Classic), *Gu Yin Liu Zi Jue* (Six Healing Sounds), *Xiao Yao Gong* (Free and Easy Exercise), *Ba Duan Jin*, *Tian Zhu Dao Yin Gong*, *Song Rou Gong* (Soft and Relaxed Exercise), *Liu He Gong* (Six-Unity Exercise) and *Fang Song Gong* (Relaxation Exercise).

The World Health Organization (WHO) defines health as "a state of complete physical, mental, and social well-being and not merely the absence of disease or infirmity." To address the unprecedented health challenges of infectious diseases, chronic diseases, aging and mental health issues, the WHO is seeking low-cost interventions to reduce economic burden. One of the WHO's strategic goals is to promote universal health coverage by integrating traditional and complementary medicine services into health service delivery and self-care.

In 2016, the Taiji Health Center was established within the Shanghai University of Traditional Chinese Medicine and Shanghai Academy of Traditional Chinese Medicine. The Center focuses on Taiji, aims to help achieve health as "a state of complete physical, mental, and social well-being", and thus constructs a self-healing Taiji health model by combining ancient health preservation, Daoyin, massage, food therapy, herbal diet and mental regulation. Professor Li Jie and her colleagues compiled another five books (in Chinese and English) on health preservation: *Zhu Bing Yuan Hou Lun Dao Yin* Shu (Daoyin Recorded in Zhu Bing Yuan Hou Lun), *Zhan Zhuang Gong* (Post Standing Exercise), *Xing Bu Gong* (Qigong Exercise in Walking), *Wo Gong* (Qigong Exercise in Lying Position) and *Shen Qi Wu Xing Cao* (Exercise of Five Elements).

I firmly believe that the publication of this book series will benefit the inheritance of traditional Chinese culture and promote the public health and wellness. I deeply hope that they will continue to dedicate and make efforts to introduce excellent Chinese culture and traditional health preservation exercise to more people around the world.

Hu Hongyi
August, 2022

前 言

Preface

中华文化源远流长，历经数千年发展。中华传统养生术是其重要的组成部分，是中华民族的瑰宝，是修身治学的根本大道，是中华民族最早用以防治疾病、养生保健的重要方法之一，为人民健康做出了巨大贡献。

2015年，上海市气功研究所向海内外气功学界发出倡言——构建现代气功"气以臻道"的学术思想，同年编纂出版"中华传统经典养生术"丛书一套八种，取得良好的社会反响，在海外也取得了广泛的影响。2016年，在世界卫生组织传统医学、补充医学与整合医学部指导下，上海中医药大学成立太极健康中心，以中华传统文化之"太极"为标志，以WHO倡导的身体、心理、社会适应性和道德的完好状态为健康目标，以传统中医养生、气功、导引、按跷、食疗、药膳、心理为技术手段，结合中华太极文化的深厚底蕴，构建"太极健康"自我疗愈模式，推广和提升世界各族人民的健康与福祉。

中华传统经典养生术是"太极健康"自我身心锻炼的重要技术方法，我们在第一批出版基础上，精选编纂第二批"中华传统经典养生术"一套五种功法，涉及人的行、立、坐、卧各种姿势的锻炼方法。希望在已经到来的全球化、人口老龄化时代中，探索出一种集自我保健、疗愈与康复于一体的新型健康促进模式，构建"太极健康"的理念与平台，为当代人的身心健康服务。

上海市气功研究所
2022年夏

Traditional Chinese culture has a long-standing and well-established history of thousands of years. As an important part of it, traditional Chinese health cultivation is a treasure of the Chinese nation and the fundamental way to cultivate one's body and mind. It is also one of the earliest important methods used for disease prevention and treatment as well as life cultivation, thus making great contributions to people's health.

In 2015, Shanghai Qigong Research Institute advocated the concept of "*Qi-Dao Harmony*" for its academic advance. The *(Chinese-English) Traditional and Classical Chinese Health Cultivation* series of eight books published in the same year has achieved positive social feedback and extensive influence overseas. In 2016, under the guidance of the WHO Traditional, Complementary and Integrative Medicine (TCI) Unit, Shanghai University of Traditional Chinese Medicine (SHUTCM) established the Taiji Health Center. The center aims for the health concept advocated by WHO, which is a state of complete physical, mental and social well-being as well as moral integrity. With the traditional Chinese concept "Taiji" as its symbol, the center combines with the profound Chinese Taiji culture. It also takes traditional Chinese medicine (TCM) as the technical means, including TCM health cultivation, Daoyin, massage, dietary therapy, medicated diet, mental therapy, and so on. We hope to build a self-healing model of "Taiji Health" for the health and well-being of people all over the world.

Traditional and classical Chinese health cultivation exercises are important methods of "Taiji Health" mind-body exercises. On the basis of the first series, we have selected and compiled five kinds of exercises in the second series of *Traditional and Classical Chinese Health Cultivation*, involving exercise methods in different positions of walking, standing, sitting and lying. In this age of globalization and population aging, we try to explore a new health promotion model integrating self-care, self-healing and self-recovery, and construct the concept and platform of "Taiji Health", in order to improve the physical and mental health of contemporary people.

Shanghai Qigong Research Institute
Summer 2022

编写说明

Words from the Compilers

近年来,随着太极健康在海内外各地的逐渐传播,运用传统太极哲学、太极文化来指导人们的身心康养,促进当代人健康理念的提升以及与之相伴的各种太极健康技法,如气功、导引、太极拳、养生术等,越来越受到人们的广泛关注。中华传统养生术根植于中华传统哲学、中医学和养生学,充分发挥主动锻炼、身心调节的优势,已经越来越引起世人的广泛关注。

2016年以来,中国、希腊、西班牙、法国、日本等地先后涌现了各类太极健康机构,传播相关的太极健康理念与技法。但总体而言,海内外市场上还是缺乏太极健康的相关书籍出版,尤其没有成套、成系列的科普作品,更缺乏汉英对照的专业著作。

上海中医药大学太极健康中心、上海市气功研究所研究人员在前期研究工作基础上,继编纂出版第一批"中华传统经典养生术"取得良好反响后,此次精选编纂第二批一套五种。从历史源流、功法理论、特色要领、图解动作、分解说明与具体运用等方面进行编纂,由上海中医药大学中医英语专业人员进行翻译,并邀请专家进行中文审稿,邀请马耳他大学中医中心主任Charles Savona Ventura博士审定英文翻译。

本套丛书沿袭第一批图文并茂、视频摄像的形式,同时配以二维码,以便读者扫码观看,方便学习与传播,尤其适合海外太极健康爱好者用汉英双语来学习。

编者

As the concept of Taiji health has spread at home and abroad in recent years, people pay more attention to the traditional Taiji philosophy and Taiji culture due to their guidance on health, as well as various Taiji health techniques such as qigong, Daoyin, Taijiquan, health preservation, etc. Rooted in the traditional Chinese philosophy, traditional Chinese medicine and health preservation, traditional and classical Chinese health cultivation exercises have given full play to the advantages of active exercise and mind-body improvement, and have attracted increasing attention across the world.

Since 2016, Taiji health organizations have sprung up in China, Greece, Spain, France, Japan and other places to spread Taiji health concepts and techniques. However, there are few books related to Taiji health in domestic and overseas markets, especially popular science book series. There are even fewer bilingual Chinese-English versions of these books.

Based on their previous studies and the positive feedback of the first series, research staff at the Taiji Health Center of Shanghai University of Traditional Chinese Medicine (SHUTCM) and Shanghai Qigong Research Institute compiled five traditional and classical Chinese health cultivation exercise methods as the second series. These books cover the history, theoretical foundation, characteristics and key principles, illustrated movements and application of the five exercises. Then these contents have been translated by professional translators at SHUTCM. The Chinese version was reviewed by an expert team, while the English version was reviewed by Dr. Charles Savona Ventura, the director for the Center of Traditional Chinese Medicine at the University of Malta.

In addition to illustrations and videos, QR codes are also available for readers, which is convenient especially for overseas Taiji health fans to learn.

Compilers

目 录

Table of Contents

行 步 功 ● *Xing Bu Gong* (Qigong Exercise in Walking)

History

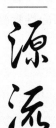

源流

行步功的源起

Origin of Qigong Exercise in Walking

气功是中国传统文化的精华内容之一，是中华民族的瑰宝，是治学修身的根本大道，也是太极健康的重要内容之一。气功的历史渊源流长，自古至今已有几千年的历史，从上古时期如4 000多年前的唐尧时期，中原地区曾洪水泛滥成灾，由于气候多雨潮湿，人们气血郁滞，易患周身及关节疼痛一类疾病，于是就用舞蹈来宣导气血以治病。《黄帝内经素问·异法方宜论》在讲述中医各种不同治法的来源时说，中原一带，平坦潮湿，人们易患肢体寒冷性疾病，或骨关节病，应该用导引按蹻来治疗。

As an essential part of traditional Chinese culture, qigong is the treasure of the Chinese nation. It is a key part of Taiji health and considered as the foundation of one's knowledge and moral character. With a time-honored history, the origin of qigong can be traced back to the era of Yao (about 4 000 years ago). At that time, the central plains were plagued by rampaging floods. Due to the rainy and humid climate, people suffered from body aches and joint pain due to qi and blood stagnation. Therefore, dances were developed to promote the circulation of qi and blood so as to alleviate pain. According to the *Huang Di Nei Jing Su Wen Yi Fa Fang Yi Lun* (Discourse on Different Therapeutic Methods for Different Diseases, the Basic Questions), people in the central plains were prone to cold limbs or joint diseases and therefore treated with Daoyin and massage.

这可以说明唐尧时期具有"宣导"作用的"舞",到春秋战国时期已发展成为医疗气功的"导引按蹻"。气功从古代传承下来又有万千流派的传承,如儒、释、道、武、医等,可以说是异彩纷呈。从功法上看有导引、吐纳、禅定、周天等,而行步功亦是气功中众多功法中的一部分。行走是人类本能的基本生命活动状态之一,古时候人们从直立、行走、奔跑以及跳跃等逐渐发展出以行走为主要形式的练功方法,形成了行步功的雏形。但行步功从古以来其名不显,并没有得到很好的推广,因为它只是散在各门各派流传的功法之中。

This indicates that "dancing" in the era of Yao had developed into Daoyin and massage that fall under the category of medical qigong. Qigong is handed down from ancient times and has been developed into five categories: Taoism, Buddhism, Confucianism, martial arts and medicine. In terms of qigong practices, there are Daoyin, breathing, meditation, and Zhou Tian Gong (microcosmic and macrocosmic orbit exercises). Qigong exercise in walking is a common exercise. Walking is an instinctive life activity of human beings. Ancient people learned to stand, walk, run and jump and finally developed a walking-oriented practicing method, which is the prototype of the qigong exercise in walking. However, the qigong exercise in walking has not enjoyed good popularity, as it is only a common qigong practice of various qigong schools.

比如据古籍记载,张家山汉简《引书》有"早起……步足堂下""却步三百而休""禹步以利股间"等。道家《抱朴子》谓:"夫导引不在于立名众物,粉绘表形著图,但无名状也,或伸屈,或俯仰,或行卧,或倚立,或躑躅,或徐步,或吟,或息,皆导引也。"又如《太清道林摄生论》谓:"人食毕,当行步踌躇,有所修为为快也""人不得夜食,食毕但当行步"。医典《诸病源候论》中说:"先行一百二十步,多者千步,然后食之。"又如《尊生要旨》:"以足相纽而行,前进十数步,后退十数步,可以祛两足风湿之邪。"

For instance, the *Yin Shu* (Book of Daoyin) unearthed at the Han tomb in Zhangjiashan states, "Get up early... Walk around the yard" "Walk 300 steps before stopping" and "Practice Yu Step (a type of qigong exercise in walking developed by King Yu in ancient times) to strengthen the hips." *Bao Pu Zi* states, "Daoyin is not limited to routine movements and can be practiced by stretching, bending, walking, lying, standing, leaning, stepping, strolling, chanting, breathing, etc." *Tai Qing Dao Lin She Sheng Lun* (Supreme Clarity Method on Health Cultivation) states, "After eating food, it is advisable to take a relaxed walk to feel comfortable and happy." "People should avoid eating at night, and if doing so, one should take a walk after eating." *Zhu Bing Yuan Hou Lun* (Treatise on Causes and Manifestations of Various Diseases) states, "Before the meal, one should walk for 120 steps or a thousand steps if possible." *Zun Sheng Yao Zhi* (Essentials for Health Cultivation) states, "Walk by taking a few dozen steps forward then a few dozen steps backward. This practice can remove wind and resolve dampness in the feet."

另外佛家也有行禅(又称经行)。可见行步功自古就有,只是隐藏在各家功法之中而大家知道的不多。行步功首次被大众所熟知则当属郭林新气功的广泛推广和传播,使得我们对行步功功法有了一个全新的认识。

Meanwhile, Buddhists have the tradition of walking meditation (also known as Jing Xing). Qigong exercise in walking has a long history but is little known by common people. Qigong exercise in walking is later known by us thanks to the popularity and dissemination of Guo Lin qigong.

华佗创立五禽戏

Hua Tuo Devised Wu Qin Xi
(Five Animal Frolics)

气功的发展从春秋以降，渐渐发展出如导引、存思、吐纳等各种方法，而五禽戏是中国传统导引养生的一个重要功法，是古代导引术的首个典型代表。其创编者华佗（约公元145—208），出生在东汉末沛国谯县（今安徽亳州）。其一生著述颇丰，但均亡佚。今传《中藏经》《华佗神医秘传》等皆托名之作。华佗弟子中著名者有吴普、樊阿、李当之等人。其中，吴普著有《吴普本草》，李当之著有《李当之药录》，而樊阿则擅长针灸及养生，据传他活到100多岁。

Since the Spring and Autumn period, qigong exercises have included Daoyin, inward contemplation, breathing, etc. Wu Qin Xi (Five Animal Frolics) is an important exercise of Daoyin. Its founder, Hua Tuo (about BC 145–BC 208), was born at Qiao county (located at Bozhou, Anhui province) in the late Eastern Han Dynasty (AD 25–AD 220). He wrote a lot of books but unfortunately these books were lost. Today's *Zhong Zang Jing* (Huatuo's Central Treasury Classic) and *Hua Tuo Shen Yi Mi Chuan* (Secret Formulas of Hua Tuo) were not written by him. Among his famous students, Wu Pu wrote *Wu Pu Ben Cao* (Wu Pu's Materia Medica), Li Dangzhi wrote *Li Dangzhi Yao Lu* (Li Dangzhi's Herbal Record) and Fan E (AD 164–AD 272) was good at acupuncture, moxibustion and health cultivation, who lived up to over 100 years according to legends.

华佗继承了前人的导引术，同时根据自己的中医理论基础，创编了较为完善的五禽戏，世人将其称为"华佗五禽戏"。华佗五禽戏的传人们都认为,其起源可以追溯到远古时代。据史料记载,当时中原大地江河泛滥,湿气弥漫,不少人患了关节不利之症。在这种情况下,古人想出了"乃制为舞""以利导之"的锻炼方法。这种意在模仿飞禽走兽动作神态的"舞",也正是远古中华气功导引术的一种萌芽。《庄子》中曾这样描写:"吐故纳新,熊经鸟伸,为寿而已矣。"这其中的"熊经鸟伸",就是对古代养生之士模仿动物姿势习练气功的描写。

Based on the predecessors' Daoyin and his own TCM theories, Hua Tuo devised Wu Qin Xi, which is later called Hua Tuo Wu Qin Xi (Huatuo's Five Animal Frolics). Its successors believed that its origin could be traced back to the time of antiquity. According to historical records, the central plains were plagued with floods and humidity. Due to the rainy and humid climate, people suffered from joint pain. At this circumstance, the ancient people invented dancing to circulate qi and blood. Such dancing was developed by imitating the postures and movements of animals and birds, which can be seen as the cradle of traditional Chinese qigong Daoyin. The *Zhuang Zi* states, "Exhale the old and inhale the new, walk like a bear and stretch the neck like a bird to achieve longevity". The "walking like a bear and stretching like a bird" is a vivid description of ancient people imitating animal postures and movements.

华佗曾对弟子吴普说:"人体欲得劳动,但不当使极耳,动摇则俗气得消,血脉流通,病不得生,户枢不朽也。"华佗继承和发展了前人"圣人不治已病治未病"的预防理论,为年老体弱者编排了一套模仿猿、鹿、熊、虎等五种禽兽姿态的养生功法——"五禽戏"。一称虎戏,二称鹿戏,三称熊戏,四称猿戏,五称鸟戏,也可以用来防治疾病,同时可使腿脚轻便利索,用来当作"气功"。身体不舒服时,就起来做其中一戏,流汗浸湿衣服后,接着在上面搽上爽身粉,身体便觉得轻松便捷,腹中想吃东西了。他的学生吴普施行这种方法锻炼，活到九十多岁时，听力和视力都很好，牙齿也完整牢固。五禽戏的动作是模仿虎的扑动前肢、鹿的伸转头颈、熊的伏倒站起、猿的脚尖纵跳、鸟的展翅飞翔等。相传华佗在许昌时，天天指导许多瘦弱的人在旷地上做这个体操。

Hua Tuo once told his student Wu Pu, "The human body needs exercise, but not excessive. When the body moves, the water and grain in the stomach can be digested, blood and qi can flow smoothly, and thus disease will not arise." Hua Tuo imitated the movements of apes, deer, bears, tigers and birds to devise Wu Qin Xi for the old and the weak by inheriting and developing predecessors' theory of "the sages usually help people prevent diseases rather than treat the diseases afterwards". Just as its name implies, Wu Qin Xi can be classified into movements of apes, deer, bears, tigers and birds. Such physical exercise can be practiced as an exercise of qigong to cure diseases and strengthen the body. When ancient people felt uncomfortable, they did this exercise. After sweating, they applied talcum powder and felt much better with an appetite for food. By practicing such exercise, Wu Pu lived to more than 90 years old with good hearing and listening, along with strong, healthy teeth. The movements of Wu Qin Xi imitated the tigers' springing forward their fore limbs, deer turning their head and neck, bears sinking down and then standing up, apes jumping with their toes and birds flying with wings spreading. According to legends, Huo Tuo often instructed people with a weak body constitution to do such exercise every day in Xuchang city.

华佗创立了五禽戏模仿各种动物形态，也是行步功法的主要来源之一。

Hua Tuo devised Wu Qin Xi by imitating animals' movements,

which later became a main source of qigong exercise in walking
exercises.

憨山大师修经行

Walking Meditation Practiced by Master Han Shan

　　汉代以后,随着佛教的传入与兴盛,许多佛教的思想和修行
方法渐渐传入中国,与中国的传统文化思想和养生修炼文化渐
渐融合,形成佛家气功的修行文化,并一直广泛流传至今。而佛
家经行即是其中一种修行方法。相传明代憨山大师二十八岁
时,有一次来到河北的盘山,山上一个茅篷里住着一位修行的老
僧,憨山大师去看他。那位老僧看见憨山来,并不理会,继续修
行。到晚上吃饭了,老僧自己做饭自己就吃了,憨山见老僧吃饭
不理他,就自己拿碗吃饭,老僧也不理他。第二天,憨山就到晚
饭时自己洗米做饭,老僧回来不说话就吃,憨山也跟着吃。每天
晚上,老僧都会到盘山顶上经行,双手甩开,大步一圈一圈地走,
憨山也跟着他一圈一圈地走。某天晚上正在经行,憨山突然好
像身心都空了,如同看见大海,整个世界都在一片光明之中,非
常的舒服清凉,此时没有杂念妄想。老僧这时已经知道了,就故
意问他:"怎么样?"憨山回答说:"一片光明中。"根据《华严经》
所述,这种境界叫"海印发光三昧"。老僧说:"这有什么了不
起,我住山三十年,夜夜经行都在这个境界里。"所以这个老僧
很了不起,这种境界不是只有打坐才能达到,站着、经行、睡觉都
可以入定,才是可贵的修行。

　　Since the introduction and popularity of Buddhism after
the Han dynasty (BC 202–AD 220), many Buddhism thoughts
and exercises have been integrated with traditional Chinese
culture and health cultivation exercises, thus forming the
Buddhism qigong. Walking meditation is a form of Buddhism
exercise. According to legend, the 28-year-old Master Han Shan
in the Ming Dynasty (AD1368–AD1644) once came to Mount

Panshan in Hebei province to visit an old monk who lived in a hut. However, when he arrived, he was totally ignored by the old monk who continued his exercise without showing any hospitality. During supper time, the old monk cooked for himself and ate without talking to Han Shan. Such being the case, Han Shan served himself. The old monk stayed silent. In the next day, Han Shan made supper and the old monk came back and ate it without saying a word. Every night, the old monk practiced walking meditation at the peak of Mount Panshan. He walked in circles with swinging arms. Han Shan just followed him walking. One night, during the walking meditation, Han Shan suddenly felt that both his body and mind were empty, as if he saw the sea and the world was bathed in the light. Without a trace of distracting thoughts, he felt very comfortable and cool. The old monk noticed and asked on purpose: "How are you feeling now?" Han Shan answered: "In a light." According to the *Hua Yan Jing* (Avatamsaka Sutra, a Buddhist classic), this state is called "Sea-illuminating meditation". The old monk continued: "This is not a big deal. I have lived here for about thirty years and experienced such status every night during walk meditation." The old monk was marvelous as he could enter meditation while controlling his mind and heart by standing, walking and sleeping, which is a valuable exercise.

八卦掌的传说
——武术气功中的行步功

Legend of Ba Gua Zhang (Eight-Diagram Palm): Qigong Exercise in Walking within Martial Arts

八卦掌是中华民族传统武术中的一份珍贵遗产，它不仅是一套高超的防身技艺,更是一种老幼咸宜、雅俗共赏的健身功法。它是内外双修的拳术,是一种以掌法变换和行步走转走圈为主的拳术。它结合了道家的导引吐纳术,融技击、养生、健身于一体,讲究内外相合、上下相随、以意领气、以气领力,可以强身健体,而且能够锻炼攻防搏击的技能。也有人认为八卦掌本来是南方道家炼丹修道之士,为了养性修身所研创的功法,向无外传。这种拳术将攻防招数和导引方法融合于绕圆走转之中。讲求纵横交错,随走随练,以变应变,合于《周易》中"刚柔相摩、八卦相荡",即运动不息,变化不止的道理,故名。

Ba Gua Zhang (Eight-Diagram Palm) is a precious legacy of traditional Chinese martial arts. It is not only an efficient self-defending technique, but also a health-benefiting exercise for the elder and the young. It emphasizes the cultivation of internal qi and physical exercise, featuring palm changes and footwork. Ba Gua Zhang combines Daoyin and breathing of Taoism with combating, health cultivation and bodybuilding. It combines the internal and external, uses the intent to guide qi and uses qi to guide strength. Practicing Ba Gua Zhang can strengthen our bodies and improve our combating skills. Some people believe that it originated from the secretive health cultivation exercise developed by Taoists who combined attack and defending movements as well as Daoyin with walking in circles. It can be practiced anytime and the movements can adapt to circumstances. The exercise is in line with the theory of "combination of softness and strength and overlapping eight diagrams" in the *Yi Jing* (Book of Changes), and therefore, it was named "Ba Gua Zhang".

八卦掌自祖师董海川创建至今,已有160多年的历史。董海川生于清嘉庆二年(1797年),逝于光绪八年(1882年),原名董明魁,清代河北文安朱家务村人。清道光三十年(1850年)前后，董海川来北京城，投身肃王府当差，董海川因多年习武，常在夜晚无人时练功，后被王府总管全凯亭发现。全凯亭略懂武功，有意经常接触董海川，但几次靠近董海川都没成功，才知董海川武功深厚。一次在肃王庆贺寿日集会之时，组织武术表演与比试。董海川当时负责肃王茶差，而比武场又被王公大臣家眷围得水泄不通。此时肃王要茶水，董海川无法入内，情急之下，便腾空跃起，从众人头上越过，来到肃王面前献茶。这一举动惊动了在场所有人员，肃王命其献艺，董海川演示了自己创编的转掌，即八卦掌，在场的武林高手无不惊讶。

Ba Gua Zhang was established by Master Dong Haichuan, with a history spanning more than 160 years. Dong Haichuan (1797–1882), whose former name was Dong Mingkui, was born in Zhujiawu village, Wen'an county, Hebei province. Around 1850, he came to the capital city Beijing and found a job in the palace of Prince Su (1866–1922). He used to practice kung fu at night when there was no one around. Later his practice was noticed by the housekeeper Wang Kaiting who knew kung fu. Wang wanted to test Dong's capability but failed a few times and realized his high skill in martial arts. Once Prince Su organized a competition of martial arts at his birthday assembly, Dong was responsible for serving tea. At that time Prince Su ordered tea, but Dong could not approach him and perform the duty due to the crowd. Under this circumstance, he had no choice but to jump across the crowd and pour tea for Prince Su, which shocked the guests present. Then Prince Su asked him to perform his martial arts. Dong showed the audience Ba Gua Zhang devised by himself and amazed the audience.

于是，肃王任命董海川为王府武术总教师，京城武林为之震动，比武者络绎不绝。董海川此时在北京首传八卦掌，凡与董海川比武者均败北。后来，号称杨无敌的杨露禅先生与董海川比武后表示，自己与董海川比武只能比个平手，胜董海川很难。两人武术的修为，让他们成为好友。当时在善扑营任教头的尹福经人介绍与董海川比武，只一手尹福即败北，立即磕头拜师，从此董海川名声大震。此后，人们都管他叫董祖师，他开武术界先河，取依圆走转、变换掌势之法，创出八卦掌的雏形"转掌"，并开始传授门徒。董祖师所传掌势经后人"复安易理，定八卦合五行加添招数，代代相传"，遍布各地，形成武术一大门派。董祖师因材施教，各授其技，为后来八卦掌形成不同风格奠定了基础，也为八卦掌的传播作出了贡献。

Then Prince Su appointed him as the kung fu master of his palace, which shocked the martial arts professionals in Beijing. Many came to challenge Dong but all ended up in failure. Later, Yang Luchan (1799–1872), whose nickname was Yang the Unconquered, confessed that defeating Dong was very difficult. Because of their extraordinary skills in martial arts, they became good friends. Another example was Yin Fu (1840–1909), another kung fu master. He was beaten by Dong with only one round and then begged Dong to teach him martial arts. Since then, Dong had been a household name. He was respectfully referred to as "Pioneer Dong" as he created the prototype of the famous Ba Gua Zhang: palm-turning featuring footwork in circles with palm changes. He taught numerous students his self-made martial arts. Moreover, his palm movements have been enriched by the followers with knowledge from Ba Gua (Eight-Diagram) and Wu Xing (Five Elements). Dong taught different techniques of Ba Gua Zhang and laid the foundation for various Ba Gua Zhang styles and made contributions to its introduction.

八卦掌由于历代名人辈出，且风格各异，引起世人瞩目。尹福、程廷华等为八卦掌第二代传人，是八卦门中公认的成就较大、建树较高的佼佼者。这些人都是董海川的入室弟子，不过董祖师都是因材施教，因人授法，善于启发弟子从实际出发，以《易》理悟拳理，因此第二代以走为基础、以变为法度，流派纷呈，不拘一格，其中，尹福和程廷华最为有名。

Ba Gua Zhang became well known to the world thanks to its different styles and generations of masters. Yin Fu and Cheng Tinghua taught by Dong himself were the most well-learned and famous students, but their palm movements were not the same as Dong. They further developed the movements based on *Yi Jing* (Book of Changes).

程廷华生于1844年，逝于1900年，河北深县程家村人，自幼进京学徒，艺成后在北京崇文门外（哈德门）花市上四条经营一家眼镜店铺，后来江湖人称之为"眼镜程"。程廷华年轻时喜好摔跤。后投师董海川门下，经数年磨炼，程廷华深得八卦掌之精妙。他经常把董海川从肃王府接出来，到自己家中居住，随时向老师请教。后来逐步形成了自己的"游身八卦连环掌"，这套掌法行云流水，连绵不断，动如猛虎，静如泰山，变化无穷。

Cheng Tinghua (1844–1900) was born in Chengjia Village, Shen County, Hebei province. When he was a little boy, he was sent to Beijing to be an apprentice to make eyeglasses. After he acquired the workmanship, he started to run a shop to sell eyeglasses on a busy street named Chongwen Men (or Hade Gate). For this reason, people also nicknamed him "Glasses Cheng". When he was young, he liked wrestling. Later on, he learned from Dong and acquired the essence of Ba Gua Zhang after years of practice. He often invited Dong to his house and consulted with him on martial art questions. Later, he developed his distinct palm movements called "Swimming

Dragon Ba Gua Palm" featuring huge changes with great power.

　　程先生的箭步功夫甚大。据程家村老人讲，有一次先生回程家村，当时，本村的几个十余岁的孩子知道程先生有武功，腿快，便央求先生去村外捉野兔，当距兔十余丈时，兔突然跃起，可转瞬间野兔却已在先生手中，而未有人得见程先生是怎样过去的。实际上先生是用箭步擒兔，可见其腿功之快。董海川去世后，这一支脉就成了后来影响极大的"程式游身八卦掌"。当初董海川年老以后，他经常坐视指导，多由程廷华代师教授，故此程式八卦掌传播得比较广泛。程式八卦掌的后人孙禄堂于1916年著有《八卦掌学》一书，孙锡堃则于1934年著《八卦掌真传》，这些书籍把八卦掌这门神奇的武术保留了下来。

Cheng is highly skillful in Jian Bu (sudden stride forward). According to the villagers, when he came back to his village, some teenagers begged him to catch rabbits. Although they knew he was fast, to their surprise Cheng could seize a rabbit more than 30 meters away in a blink. In fact, this attributed to Cheng's great strides. When Dong grew old, he asked Cheng to perform the teaching movements as instructed. Since he passed away, Cheng's Swimming Dragon Ba Gua Palm has been one of the most popular Ba Gua Zhang branches. Among Cheng's followers, Sun Lutang (1860–1933) and Sun Xikun wrote books on Ba Gua Zhang in 1916 and 1934 correspondingly, which contributed to reserve Ba Gua Zhang as a marvelous martial art.

　　八卦掌是中国传统武术的一大门派，八卦掌的文化实则就是中华文化的一部分，比如文极而武、武极而文就是中华阴阳哲理，中国武术不同于西方，我们的武术是一种文化，一种修身养性的方式，讲究的是修养。

As an important school of traditional Chinese martial arts,

Ba Gua Zhang is also an important part of Chinese culture. Studying culture is necessary when one is an expert on martial arts to a certain degree, while one should seek inspiration from martial arts to be more sophisticated in culture. This mutuality manifests the philosophy of yin and yang. Unlike Western combating skills, Chinese martial arts are deeply rooted in Chinese culture and emphasize self-cultivation.

　　八卦掌的理论基础是阴阳八卦理论,而这一理论在八卦掌中的应用主要是先后天八卦图分别在内修和外修中的应用,现代认为八卦掌是以含八卦之体,按先天八卦图来练对应之体内八卦,使人体诸脉畅通,内气充实,身心健康,筋骨柔韧,肌肉坚实,反应敏捷,动作迅速,劲顺力达,体能得以最大限度的应用,最终融合于大自然返先天成为无极之体。以身体之阴阳对应的格斗动作按八卦取象的八种动物练成掌式,掌握合于阴阳五行的一些技巧、方法、技术和原则,以使人在对敌实战中能以小胜大,以巧打蛮,以少胜多,同时在技击中遵循阴阳八卦的消长转化、变化无穷的原则,并严格遵循易理运转不停。

The theoretical foundation of Ba Gua Zhang originated from yin and yang and eight diagrams. Today, it is believed that practicing Ba Gua Zhang helps to match the eight-diagram within the body with the primordial eight diagrams, ensure the free flow of qi and blood to strengthen the inner qi, enable the sinews and bones to be more flexible and muscles to be firm, maintain a quick response and unleash the maximum physical potential. The eight diagrams (Eight Ba Gua-oriented-animal movements), coupled with techniques and principles of yin, yang and five elements, can genuinely defeat enemies much stronger and bigger in size.

郭林新气功
——现代行步功的倡导者

Guo Lin Qigong: Advocate of
Modern Qigong Exercise in Walking

中华人民共和国成立后,20世纪50年代,第一个提倡气功治病的人是刘贵珍(1902—1983),他于河北唐山创立气功疗养院。第二个高潮的带头人之一是郭林女士(1909—1984),她于1971年9月4日在北京的公园开始为广大群众宣传气功治病原理,说服病人跟她学练功。她常对人说的生命只有一次,当然是重要,但还有比生命更重要的,那就是人生一世,应当做一番有利于人类的事业。她的口号是"致力新气功,造福为人民"。她不取分文,义务教功,所创编的新气功能防治癌症及多种慢性病、疑难症,目前,已传播到世界多个国家。

After the founding of the People's Republic of China, the first person who advocated to cure diseases with qigong was Liu Guizhen (1902–1983), who built a sanatorium in Tangshan, Hebei province in the 1950s. The second advocate was Ms. Guo Lin (1909–1984). She lectured the principle of curing diseases with qigong to the ordinary people in Beijing parks on September 4th, 1971 and convinced the sick to follow her to practice qigong. She often said that staying alive was important, what was more important over the course of life was to help others. She taught qigong for free and her self-made Guo Lin qigong could be an auxiliary method to deal with chronic diseases. Today, her qigong has spread to many countries in the world.

郭林女士为人诚实忠厚,平易近人,履仁行义,学而不厌,诲人不倦。她亲自培育出一支素质很好的辅导员队伍,他们都是跟她学习新气功治愈的病友，自愿终生从事发展新气功，为人类健康幸福而献身于伟大事业。

Guo Lin is kind, honest and easy-going. She was insatiable in learning and tireless in teaching. She trained a team of qigong advocates, mainly composed of patients who followed her to practice qigong. As a result, they were willingly committed to advancing the undertaking of qigong and making contributions to the health and happiness of other people.

她所执着追求的是"致力新气功"要科学化，"造福为人民"要大众化。她由身患癌症经加练气功治愈后，见到不少人也患有癌症及慢性病，遂根据家传、师传的功法与自身的练功体验，对传统气功进行了改革，在功法上创编了易教、易学、易练的郭林新气功。郭林新气功问世不久，就辅助治愈了一些疑难症，包括青光眼、癌症与危重症，于是气功从以前防治功能性疾病、慢性病，发展到也可以辅助治疗一些器质性疾病。

She pursued to improve qigong in a more scientific way and to enable it to benefit more people. She combined traditional qigong exercises with her own experience to create the easy-to-learn Guo Lin qigong, which later has been proven to be helpful for glaucoma, cancer and critical conditions. Since then, qigong has become a therapy for some organic diseases, apart from some functional and chronic diseases.

目前，世界医学形势正处在微妙变化时刻，已由微观世界精细分析而要回到宏观世界系统科学方面来，已渐由偏重外因治疗逐渐转移到重视内因潜力上来。很多国家正在大力开展气功疗法研究。多年来，如对慢性病中的结核病，虽然有各种抗结核药物治疗，也是有效的，但是它还有一定的局限性和副作用。它强调了偏重外因治疗（抑制细菌），但有时治肺伤肝、治肝伤肾，顾此失彼，非尽善尽美。因此，有识医家提出"药源性疾病"之论。总之，目前单纯依靠药物对肺结核病的治疗还不够理想。

At present, the mode of global medical treatment has shifted from detailed analysis to systematic science and focused more on the treatment of internal causes over external pathogenic factors. This is why many countries endeavor to conduct research qigong therapy. For example, anti-tuberculosis drugs are effective but cause side effects, as they emphasize treating external pathogenic factors (such as inhibiting the bacteria and extinguishing the infection). This may harm our liver when curing lung diseases or harm the kidney while treating liver disorders. Therefore, knowledgeable doctors now propose the idea of drug-induced diseases or drug-caused harms. It shows that drugs alone are not enough for tuberculosis.

中医学从整体着眼，认为病之起源与病之治愈，始终不出内因和外因正邪斗争之关系。所谓"正气存内，邪不可干""邪之所凑，其气必虚""治病必求于本"。所以防治疾病强调扶正祛邪、培本清源为总的原则。练功可以调动内气，增强机体抵抗力，能使人体疾病产生的内因发生变化，可以起到药物所起不到的作用。郭林新气功理法就是强调自力更生，练出内气，自行调控治病，不主张发放外气治病。她看到世界医学形势在变化中，东西文化哲学在交流中，提出在对治癌病与疑难慢性病时，要药物治疗与气功治疗相结合，不要丢掉药物。倡导气功治病要与中医、西医相结合。这些，都推动了气功事业向前发展。

From the holistic view of Chinese medicine, the onset and recovery of disease are all associated with the struggle between healthy qi and pathogenic factors. Just as the statements of "when there is sufficient healthy qi inside, the pathogenic qi has no way to invade the body", "the accumulation of pathogens means the deficiency of healthy qi" and "seek the root cause for disease treatment" in *Huang Di Nei Jing* (Yellow Emperor's Inner Classic). Practicing qigong can activate one's internal qi and strengthen one's body resistance. This effect is better than drugs alone. The principle of Guo Lin qigong lies in cultivating one's internal qi to fight against diseases rather than relying on external qi. From the shift of global medical model and the exchange between Eastern and Western philosophy, Guo Lin proposed to combine drug treatment, TCM methods and qigong therapy for cancer and chronic diseases.

从上述行步功的简要发展历史，我们可知它们都是我们传统祛病养生健身文化的重要组成部分，至今依然在人类健康事业中发挥着重要的作用。

The brief history of qigong exercise in walking has demonstrated that it is truly an important part of traditional health culture. Today it is still playing a key role in the promotion of human health.

行步功法也可大致分为养生类和功夫类这两大类，养生类主要是以祛病养生，保持身心健康为目的，如郭林新气功、矮步行功、逍遥行步功等；而功夫类则广泛存在于各门派的各种功法之中，如形意拳、八卦掌等，特别强调腿脚的功夫。例如当代形意大师李仲轩，曾跟随唐维禄学拳，唐维禄说："形意拳又叫行意拳，有个行字，功夫正在两条腿上。"又说："你走远路来学拳，走路也是练功夫。"另外八卦转掌也特别强调一个"行"字，要两腿走的如行云流水才行。

The exercises of qigong exercise in walking can mainly be classified into two groups: health cultivation and martial arts. The former aims to cure diseases, cultivate health and keep one's body and mind healthy, including Guo Lin qigong, Bent-Leg qigong exercise in walking and Xiao Yao (free and easy) qigong exercise in walking. The latter aims to train one's legs and feet, including Xing Yi Quan (Form-Intent Fist) and Ba Gua Zhang (Eight-Diagram Palm). For example, when Xing Yi Quan master Li Zhongxuan (1905–2004) learned the martial art from Tang Weilu (1868–1944), Tang once said: "the power of Xing Yi Quan rests on one's legs." He also said, "you walked to learn fist exercise, walking is also a way of practicing kung fu." Besides, Ba Gua Zhang also puts its stress on walking in a fast and smooth way.

为了让大家更好地学习与研究行步功法，我们编撰这本《行步功》，辑录了一些很有代表性的行步功法，既有养生类也有功夫类，希望进一步丰富太极健康的气功功法，也为广大气功爱好者的健康做出一定的贡献。

I wrote this book for readers to better study the exercises of qigong exercise in walking, including both health cultivation and martial arts exercises. I sincerely hope this can further enrich qigong exercises of Taiji Health and benefit the health of qigong fans.

行 步 功 • *Xing Bu Gong* (Qigong Exercise in Walking)

Theoretical Foundation

理
论
基
础

气功是中国传统祛病养生的重要方法之一，在其长期发展过程中，不断融合中华古代传统的哲学与思想，形成了自身独特的理论与学说。行步功作为气功的一部分，也有自己的基本理论，特别是与练功三调和内炼精气神有紧密的关联。

Qigong is a traditional way of curing diseases and cultivating health in China. Over its development, it has formed its unique theory by absorbing traditional Chinese philosophy and ideology. As a part of qigong, qigong exercise in walking also has its own theory, which is closely associated with the three regulations and internal exercise of essence, qi and spirit.

练功三调
Three Regulations

具有悠久历史的气功养生锻炼，与其他锻炼方法相比有非常独特的特点，就是其最大的技术手段为三调和三调合一。

The most distinctive characteristics of the time-honored qigong exercise are three regulations (body regulation, breath regulation and mind regulation) and their unity.

调身是调控身体的姿势或运动的动作活动，也称炼形、身法等。调身在于使身体的状态与练功所要求的境界相应。例如练静功时身体须保持某一固定的姿势，这与进入静定的气功境界相应；而练动功则多与疏通经络、调动内气运行的气功境界相应，以外动导引内气。

Body regulation, also called body adjusting, refers to the regulation of body postures and movements. It requires matching the status of body with the purpose of practice. For instance, when practicing static qigong, one should keep a fixed posture which matches the status of static qigong; dynamic qigong practice usually matches the purposes of unblocking meridians, activating internal qi and guiding the internal qi by external movements.

调息是调控呼吸的活动，也称炼气，又称吐纳等。调息在于通过调控呼吸而孕育和引导内气，是练功进入气功境界的重要方法。一吸一呼为一息，其中尤以呼气与内气密切相关，内气多随呼气而生发运行。此外，现代研究已证明，调息可以调节自主神经系统中交感神经和副交感神经的张力，从而可以调整相应的内脏组织器官的功能。调息的内容包括两个方面，一是呼吸形式的调控，即进行自然呼吸、腹式呼吸等不同呼吸形式的操作。二是出入气息的调控，使之或强或弱，或粗或细。这两个方面互相关联、相互作用，呼吸形式的改变可以引导气息出入的变化，反之亦然。

Breath regulation, also called refining qi or breathing, refers to the regulation of one's breath. As an important part of qigong practice, it aims to generate and guide more internal qi. Breathing consists of exhaling and inhaling and the latter is closely linked to the generation of internal qi. Moreover, modern studies have proven that breathing regulation can regulate the tension of sympathetic nerves and parasympathetic nerve in the vegetative nervous system, thus adjusting corresponding functions of internal organs and tissues. Breath regulation includes regulating breathing patterns such as natural breathing and abdominal breathing as well as the strength of breathing to make it stronger or weaker. These two aspects are interconnected and mutually affect each other. Therefore, the changes of breathing patterns can alter the strength of breathing and vice versa.

调心是调控精神心理状态的活动,也称炼神等。调心在于改变日常意识活动的内容和方式,进入气功境界所需要的意识状态。一般日常生活中的意识活动属外向性,练气功则需要将意识活动转为内向,导致了意识活动内容和方式的变化。

Mind regulation, also called spirit-refining, refers to the regulation of one' mental and psychological state. It aims to change the content and pattern of conscious activities so as to help one enter the conscious state required in qigong practice. Generally speaking, one's conscious activities in daily life focus on the outside world, while practicing qigong turns them into concentrating on the inner, which causes the changes in the content and pattern of conscious activities.

三调(调身、调息、调心)是学练气功的基本操作内容,三调合一则构成气功境界。故学练气功仅仅学习三调操作还不够,还必须懂得和把握三调合一。学练之初,常用的方法是首先逐一学习三调操作的内容,将每一调的操作内容分别掌握至熟练。在本质上,气功修炼中的三调本来就不曾分离,调心、调息、调身是统一练功过程中有机联系在一起的三个方面、三种角度。随着三调的操作不断深入和熟练,三调之间的界限会越来越模糊,而它们之间的有机联系和协同性会日益显现,最终成为练功境界发展的主导力量,三调合一便会自然到来。三调合一也可以从其中的任何一调入手,将其操作至极致,就会自然地吸引、吸收其他两调,从而达到一调中包含三调,三调融合为一调的气功境界。

Three regulations (body regulation, breath regulation

and mind regulation) are basic elements of practicing qigong. The unity of the three is the prerequisite of qigong. In other words, it's not enough to learn three regulations but to unite the tree into one. In order to reach that level, one needs to first command the movements of each regulation. In essence, the three regulations are never separable and they are interrelated three aspects or perspectives in the practice of qigong exercise. When one becomes skillful at the three regulations, the boundaries among them will become indistinct. On the contrary, they are more and more interconnected and eventually become the driving force of advanced qigong practice. Alternatively, one can start with the proficiency of one regulation and then gradually extend to the other two regulations, integrating three regulations into one.

行步功作为气功养生术的一部分，也特别强调三调和三调合一，它以行走为主要练功形式，从调身入手，渐渐的结合调心与调息，最后达到三调合一的高级境界。

As a part of qigong health cultivation, qigong exercise in walking stresses on the three regulations and their unity. It uses walking as the main form of exercise and starts with body regulation, then gradually integrates breath and mind regulations and achieves the advanced level in qigong practice: the unity of the three regulations.

内炼精气神
Internal Exercise of Essence, Qi and Spirit

在古往今来各门各派的传统养生健身文化中，内炼精气神都是其中最核心的内容养生，主要养的就是人的"精、气、神"。古代养生家遵循正确的修炼方法，往往能够获得健康和高寿。

Internal exercise of essence, qi and spirit is the foundation in all schools of health cultivation. The key is to cultivate essence, qi and spirit. Ancient scholars who highlighted health cultivation could obtain health and longevity through correct exercise methods.

精、气、神本是古代哲学中的概念，是指形成宇宙万物的原始物质，含有元素的意思。中医认为精、气、神是人体生命活动的根本。在古代讲究养生的人，都把"精、气、神"称为人身的三宝，所以保养精、气、神是健身、延缓衰老的主要原则，尤其是当精、气、神逐渐衰退变化，人已步入老年的时候就更应该珍惜此"三宝"。

Originally, essence, qi and spirit were philosophical concepts, referring to the primordial matter or elements that formed all things in the universe. In Chinese medicine, essence, qi and spirit are the material foundation for vital activities. Ancient people who highlighted health cultivation considered essence, qi and spirit as three treasures of the body. Evidently, the main principle to stay healthy, nurture life and delay aging is to preserve essence, qi and spirit, especially for the elderly with gradual decline in these three treasures.

"精"就是指人体一切精微物质。有先后天之分。先天之精就是指元精，包括生殖之精（包含遗传信息的物质）。元精是人体生长发育的基础物质，它来自父母的精血，是构成人体生命活动的原始精微物质，元精随着人体生长发育，逐渐产生生殖之精。后天之精主要包括五脏六腑内所贮藏的精华物质，血液、津液和各种内分泌液等。气功锻炼能使先天和后天之精逐渐充养，就能提高人体精力和生殖能力。

Essence is the nutrient substance of life. Congenital essence refers to primordial essence or reproductive essence inherited from one's parents (including genetic information), i.e., material foundation for human growth and development. Acquired essence refers to essential nutrients stored in five-zang and six-fu organs, including blood, body fluids and endocrine secretions. Qigong practice can supplement both congenital and acquired essence and thus improve one's vigor and reproductive capacity.

"气"就是指人体的生命力，也可以理解为生命运行的能量，也有先天后天之分。先天之气就是指元气，又叫原气、真气，古代常称"炁"。所谓元气可理解为人体的生命力、免疫力、康复力，就是人体生命活动的动力。后天之气主要包括五脏六腑的功能活动，经络系统的功能活动和具有温养功能的卫气，以及具有营养成分的营气等。因此，气功锻炼能使先后天之气逐渐充足，就能增强人体的免疫功能和生理功能。对提高体力、增强体质、养生保健、延缓衰老尤为重要。

Qi is the vital energy of life. Congenital qi, also known as *Yuan*-primordial qi or *Zhen*-genuine qi, can be understood as human vitality, immunity or recuperative ability. Acquired qi includes functional activities of zang-fu organs and meridians, *Wei*-defense qi that warms and defends the body and *Ying*-nutrients qi that nurtures the body. Qigong exercise can gradually supplement acquired qi, boost the physiological functions and immune system and thus increase the body constitution, promote health and delay aging.

"神"就是人体意识、思维和智慧，与心和脑的关系最为密切。中医认为"心藏神""脑为元神之府"。神有先后天之分。先天之神就是指元神，可以理解为一种最原始的灵性。后天之神就是指识神，指通过各种学习以后所获得的知识、感觉和思辨能力。所以，养生气功锻炼能使先后天之神逐渐旺盛，就能养成良好的心态，调节心理功能，提高大脑功能，对开发智力、发挥潜能、改善睡眠、增强记忆、预防痴呆等有较好作用。

Spirit refers to mental consciousness, thought and wisdom. It is closely associated with the heart and brain. In Chinese medicine, the heart stores spirit and the brain houses spirit. Congenital spirit refers to primordial spirit. Acquired spirit refers to knowledge perception and critical thinking ability through learning. Qigong exercise can supplement acquired spirit, cultivate a good mental state, regulate emotions, develop intelligence, improve sleep, increase memory and prevent dementia.

中国传统养生修炼文化特别讲究内炼精气神，其阶次一般可分为筑基、炼精化气、炼气化神、炼神还虚几个阶段。元代陈致虚《金丹大要》卷四曰："是皆不外神气精三物，是以三物相感，顺则成人，逆则生丹。何为顺？一生二，二生三，三生万物，故虚化神，神化气，气化精，精化形，形乃成人。何谓逆？万物含三，三归二，二归一，知此道者怡神守形，养形炼精，积精化气，炼气合神，炼神还虚，金丹乃成。"

Internal exercise of essence, qi and spirit is vital in internal alchemy. The cultivation process can be divided into four stages: construction of the foundations, refining essence to qi, refining qi to spirit and refining spirit back to emptiness. *Jin Dan Da Yao* (The Great Essentials of the Golden Alchemy) written by Chen Zhixu in the Yuan Dynasty (1271–1368) states, "There are only three things: spirit, qi, and essence. The three things are interconnected; if you follow them, you may create lives; if you oppose them, you may cultivate the elixir. What does 'follow' mean? One produced two, two produced three, and three produced all things, so the emptiness turns into spirit, spirit turns into qi, qi turns into essence, essence turns into form, and form makes lives. What does 'oppose' mean? Everything contains three, three contains two, and two contains one. Those who are aware of this knowledge can guard their spirit, cultivate their body to refine essence, accumulate essence to transform qi, refine qi with spirit, refine the spirit back to emptiness, and thus form the golden elixir."

中国养生学乃至中国哲学，主张的是神物一元的，即统合于太极大道，并不存在意识和物质的绝对对立。"神物"之间，由"气"来统一为一体。精、气、神，构成中国传统养生和生命学说的重要组成部分。《太平经》说："神者受之于天，精者受之于地，气者受之于中和。"三者统一于气，并互相增强和促进。通过行气导引的方法，如一般人可以通过合理运动、气功练习，道家通过内丹修炼，佛家通过静坐禅定等方法，来增强元气，进一步促进化生精、神，达到精气神的统一和圆满，成就养生的最高境界。

From the perspective of Chinese philosophy and health cultivation, spirit and essence attribute oneness. In other words, spirit and essence are united by qi. These three treasures play a key role in life theory and traditional Chinese health cultivation. The *Tai Ping Jing* (The Scripture on Great Peace) states, "Spirit is endowed by the heaven, essence by the earth and qi by harmony". For ordinary people, *Yuan*-primordial qi can be supplemented by appropriate exercise and qigong practice. For Daoist priests, *Yuan*-primordial qi can be supplemented by internal alchemy. For Buddhist monks, *Yuan*-primordial qi can be supplemented by meditation. All these methods can promote, transform and generate essence, qi and spirit and accomplish the highest state of health cultivation.

行步功也继承了内炼精气神这一传统养生的精髓，通过行走的方式练功，日久功深，渐渐的凝练精气神，以达到健康长寿的目的。

Qigong exercise in walking also inherits the internal exercise of essence, qi and spirit. By practicing qigong through walking, one can gradually cultivate the essence, qi and spirit and thus achieve health and longevity.

行 步 功 • *Xing Bu Gong* (Qigong Exercise in Walking)

Characteristics and Essential Principles

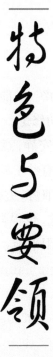

行步功作为气功养生的一部分，具有气功的基本特色和要求，也有自己特有的一些特色与要领。

Qigong exercise in walking is a part of qigong health cultivation. It has unique characteristics and essential principles.

行步功特色
Characteristics of Qigong Exercise in Walking

动静结合
Motion and Stillness

动与静是对立的统一，能够相互影响，相互促进，相互转化，二者结合有利于气功修炼。本功法在行进时练功，要求动中有静，外形运动而神意安静，意念集中，此即所谓动中寓静。故动与静的有机结合，既有益于外在的形体运动，又有益于内气的聚集与运行，能够形神兼炼，更有效地提高练功效果。行步功以行走作为主要练功形式，也很强调动静结合，心神内敛，外动而内静，以达到身心的阴阳平衡。

Body movements and inner cultivation are the unity of opposites. They interact and transform into each other. The two are both needed in qigong practice. Qigong exercise in walking is practiced through walking. It combines active body movements with inner tranquilization (mental focus). In addition, movements of qigong exercise in walking are soft but not slack, hard but not rigid. They are perfect combination of softness in hardness and hardness in softness, containing genuine qi and internal strength.

下盘沉稳
Lower Body Stability

行步功是在行走中练功，故而对下盘腿部的要求比较高，为保证练功时身体不会摇晃，要求增加腿部的实力，使下盘沉稳，也可在行步功的习练中慢慢增强下盘的实力，只有下盘沉稳了，才能逐渐延长行步的时间以及调整下盘姿势的高低。

Strengthening the lower body is necessary to maintain stability during walking. Qigong exercise in walking can gradually increase the leg strength and lay the groundwork for posture adjustments.

松柔圆活
Soft, Round and Flexible

即体松心静，这是气功锻炼的基本原则。要求动作舒展柔和，速度缓慢均匀，姿态圆活灵动，通过练功使身体肢节松软，不要僵硬死板，要"松而不懈""柔中有刚"。配合呼吸的舒畅细匀，意识的宁静祥和，以期达到调和气血，调理脏腑的作用。圆活是在练功时，躯干身体各节保持圆形，各关节不要僵直。这是依据太极圆周运行不息而来的。

A relaxed body and a tranquil mind are essential for qigong practice. Ease and roundness are essential for the body movements. Through practice, one can soften the body and joints and achieve "relaxation without flaccidity" and "hardness within softness". With natural breathing, a tranquil mind and even, unhurried and flexible movements can harmonize qi and blood and benefit the zang-fu organs. Instead of causing stiffness or rigidity, the movements of qigong exercise in walking are round, flexible, adaptable (change with ease) and uninterrupted.

循序渐进
Step by Step

循序渐进是指在行步功锻炼过程中，要根据功法的要求，认真地去做，要有毅力，需要较长时间坚持不懈的练习，并且根据自己身体的实际情况，使行走的距离渐渐延长，姿态渐渐坐低，从调身入手，结合调息，再结合调心，步步深入，层层递进，以达到三调合一进入忘形无我的气功状态。

It's important to practice qigong exercise in walking step by step — start with regulating the body, then breathing and finally the mind, so as to achieve the unity of the three regulations. It's worth noting that it takes time and efforts to achieve such level.

行步功基本身法要领
Essential Principles of Body Movements during Qigong Exercise in Walking

虚领顶劲
Hold the Head as if Suspended from Above

在行步功练习时注意略收下颌，将玉枕骨竖起。而神与气自然相遇于顶。虚领顶劲指头顶的百会穴（从两耳尖直上头顶与两耳垂连线交会处）要虚虚上领，额前天庭处略向前顶劲，颈部肌肉不是强直用力梗脖，而是略向上拉伸，要求保持颈肌有弹性，这是一种自然用劲状态。这样做有利于放松颈椎后部，改善头部的气血运行。

When practicing qigong exercise in walking, slightly tuck in the lower jaw, and keep the head upright as if the point Baihui (GV20, located at the midpoint of the line connecting the auricular apices) is being pulled from above. To do so, use intent instead of brute force. This posture can relax the back of the cervical spine and promote the circulation of qi and blood. In this way, spirit and qi will naturally meet on the vertex.

松静自然
Relaxation and Tranquility

习练时首先要从松、静、自然入手。"松"指形体方面的放松。具体来说，就是生理状态的放松，也就是不紧张，使全身机体处在松弛、舒适状态。松是一个由浅到深、由外至内的锻炼过程，通过习练使身体、呼吸、意念均慢慢进入轻松舒适的状态。"静"指思想和情绪的平稳安宁，排除杂念干扰。松与静是相辅相成的，精神上的"静"可以促使形体上的"松"，而形体上的"松"又可助于精神上的"静"，二者缺一不可。"无为自然"是指形体、呼吸、意念都要顺其自然，勿刻意追求。

The practice should start with relaxation and tranquility. The term "relaxation" refers to the relaxation of the body, so that the whole body is in a relaxed and comfortable state. It is a comfortable state achieved by practicing from shallow to deep, from the outside to the inside, through regulating the body, breathing and mind. The term "tranquility" refers to the smoothness and tranquility of thoughts and emotions without distractions. Relaxation and tranquility are complementary. The spiritual "tranquility" can promote the physical "relaxation", and vice versa.

立身中正
Keep the Body Upright

行步功的习练无论是直线行走还是转圈行走大多要求身形特别是上身中正，不能偏斜，迈步沉稳，上身轻灵松柔，两臂自然摆动，所谓形正则气顺，随着习练的日久功深，使身体气血达到下实上虚的理想状态。

Whether walking in a straight line or walking in a circle, the body should be upright. The upper body is relaxed and flexible, with two arms swinging naturally. Over time, one can get a cleansed mind and weighted (solid) body.

敛臀松腰
Tuck in the Buttocks and Relax the Waist

习练行步功时要求始终保持敛臀松腰，腰包括左右两肾和左右腰及前腰（腹部）。松腰指腰背"肾俞"和"命门"略向后送。这同样是要用意通过放松腰部来做到，等到日久功深自然能养成习惯而不用刻意来做。敛臀是指臀部稍做内收，不向后撅起，保持后臀自然收进的姿势，这样能保持身形中正而放松。

When practicing qigong exercise in walking, one should tuck in the buttocks and relax the waist. The waist region includes the left and right kidneys, the left and right waist and the front waist (abdomen). Relaxing the waist means to use the intent to relax "Shenshu (BL23)" and "Mingmen (Du4)" on the back. Tucking in the buttocks can keep the body upright and relaxed.

稳步前行
Move Steadily

习练行步功是以行走为主要练功方式，故特别强调下盘沉稳，全身要保持稳定，不能晃动，要做到迈步既轻灵又沉稳方能达到较高的水准和功用。行步功可以和站桩功相配合，以帮助增加全身的稳定性。

The body should remain stable without swaying when practicing qigong exercise in walking. This requires the strength of the lower body. Therefore, the practice can be combined with post standing exercise to help increase the stability of the body.

行 步 功 ● *Xing Bu Gong* (Qigong Exercise in Walking)

Movements

功法操作

古往今来行步功法较多，散布在各种流派之中，包括儒、释、道、武、医等各家。以下选择几种较为独特的行步功法来做介绍。

Throughout history, there have been various schools of qigong exercise in walking, including Confucianism, Buddhism, Taoism, martial arts and medicine. In this section, we will introduce several unique qigong exercises in walking.

一、矮步行功
Bent-Leg Qigong Exercise in Walking

矮步行功是一种简单而又行之有效的行步功法，来源自古代养生导引术。因此功法简单易行，随时随地都可操作，既可室内也可室外练习，故很受古人喜爱，特别适合普通人群、爱好养生人士和儒家读书人。儒家人士练功多偏向于静功，如庄子所描述的心斋、坐忘、精思入神等，但在读书和静坐之余，也会采用一些健身锻炼的方法，矮步行功因为简单易行，故经常被采用。此功法大致有高位、中位以及低位三种不同的高低姿势，适合有不同练功需求的人士习练。矮步行功强调三调合一，并且把肢体导引、站桩和静心相结合，日久功深，能起到养生健身、调理脏腑、祛病康复的功用，对高血压、糖尿病、失眠以及多种心理疾病有较好的调节作用。

Bent-Leg qigong exercise in walking is a simple and effective practice developed on the basis of ancient Daoyin movements. It is easy to learn and suitable for health cultivation. Confucianists often practice static qigong, such as meditation. However, in addition to reading and meditation, they also need some exercises. Bent-Leg qigong exercise in walking is a good choice. It can be practiced in three postures: high-position walking, middle-position walking and low-position walking. Bent-Leg qigong exercise in walking emphasizes the combination of the three regulations, and combines Daoyin, post standing exercise and meditation. Over time, this exercise can cultivate health, regulate zang-fu organs and alleviate hypertension, diabetes, insomnia and mental disorders.

预备式
Preparation Movement

两脚微并拢，自然站立，全身放松，两眼平视前方，收视返听，宁心安神（图1-1）。

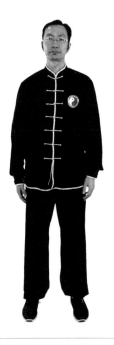

图1-1　Figure 1-1

Place the feet together. Stand naturally with a relaxed body and refreshed mind. Look straight ahead, regulate breathing and tranquilize the mind. (Figure 1–1)

操作要领
Tips

1. 调身
1. Body Regulation

（1）高位矮步行功：两膝微屈，身体缓缓下坐，膝关节尽量不超过脚尖，保持上半身正直而松，屈髋敛臀。先迈左腿，再迈右腿，保持身形高低不变，直线向前行步，两臂自然摆动，行至尽头转身往回走，可以来回转身反复行走，也可以连续转身90°折转走。（图1-2、图1-3）

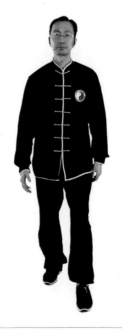
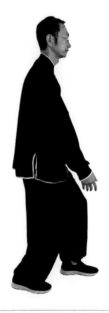

图1-2　Figure 1-2　　　　图1-3　Figure 1-3

(1) High position walking: Slightly bend the knees and do not let the knees go past the toes, keep the upper body relaxed, slightly bend the hips and tuck in the buttocks. First step the left leg and then the right leg. Keep the upper body upright and walk straight forward with two arms swinging naturally. Then turn around (either 90° or 180°) and walk back with the same requirements. (Figure 1–2 and Figure 1–3)

（2）中位矮步行功：姿势同前，唯两腿继续向下坐，达到中位站桩的高度，大腿与地面大概呈45°角，行走之时保持高度不变，锻炼时间逐渐延长。（图1–4、图1–5）

(2) Middle-position walking: Remain in the same posture as above. Slightly squat down to the middle-position post standing with an angle about 45° formed between the thighs and the ground. Keep the upper body upright when walking, and the exercise time can be extended. (Figure 1–4 and Figure 1–5)

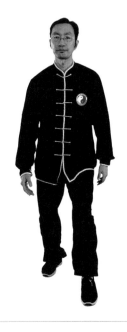

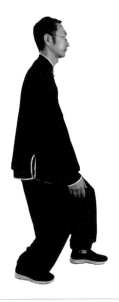

图1–4　Figure 1–4　　　　图1–5　Figure 1–5

（3）低位矮步行功：姿势同前，唯两腿继续向下坐，达到低位站桩的高度，大腿与地面接近平行，行走之时保持高度不变，锻炼时间逐渐延长。(见图1-6、图1-7)

(3) Low-position walking: Remain the same posture as above. Squat down to the low-position post standing that thighs are almost parallel to the ground. Keep the upper body upright when walking, and the exercise time can be extended. (Figure 1-6 and Figure 1-7)

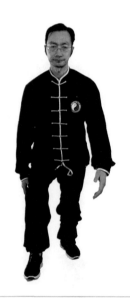 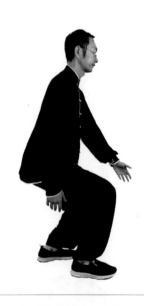

图1-6　Figure 1-6　　　　图1-7　Figure 1-7

2. 调息、调心

2. Breathing regulation and mind regulation

在练习本功法时，保持自然呼吸，同时使心神宁静并把意识专注于两脚。

When practicing, breathe naturally while calming the mind and place mental focus on the feet.

注意事项
Notes

（1）在做行功时要保持身体松静自然平稳，上身不能摇晃。同时两臂摆动要圆活自然。

(1) Keep the upper body upright and stable and let the two arms naturally swing from side to side.

（2）开始练习时以高位姿势为宜，当练习一段时间后可以逐渐坐低，但要循序渐进，以达到日久功深。

(2) It's advisable to start with the high position walking. The posture of the body can change and lower over time.

（3）当身体姿势逐渐坐低时，需要腿上有一定功力，要保持上身正直不向前倾。

(3) The strength of the legs is needed to keep the upper body upright.

（4）每次练习的时间10～30分钟，随着练功的深入逐渐延长。

(4) 10 to 30 minutes is enough for beginners. The exercise time can increase over time.

（5）习练场地要有一定的长度，可以直线转身来回行走，如空间有限，也可90°转身转圈走。

(5) To practice qigong exercise in walking, it's advisable to walk in a straight line; however, if there is not enough room, one can walk in a circle.

应用
Application

（1）中高位行功以养生祛病健身为主要功用，对高血压、糖尿病、失眠以及多种心理疾病如焦虑症、抑郁症等有较好的调节治疗作用。

(1) High-position walking and middle-position walking can help to achieve wellness and longevity and are beneficial to hypertension, diabetes, insomnia and mental disorders such as anxiety and depression.

（2）中低位行功主要是以练功夫为主，通过较长时间的练习可以强身健体，锻炼我们的筋骨皮肉和精气神，以及精神意志性格等，让身心得到全面的提升。

(2) Low-position walking is suitable for practicing martial arts. Persistent exercise can strengthen the body, exercise the muscles, bones, sinews, qi, spirit, will and character.

二、逍遥行步功
Xiao Yao (Free and Easy) Qigong Exercise in Walking

道家是中华传统文化的重要组成部分，也是古时道文化的源头之一，历时数千年延续至今，而道家气功之源可追溯到先秦之老、庄。汉以后形成的道教，使道家理论和道士的修持实践相结合，并且融合了养生家、阴阳家、医家以及巫术等其他多家的学说思想和技术方法，促进和推动了道家气功体系的发展与完善。该派功法的主要特点是强调性命双修，代表功法为内丹术，也称为"周天功"。以内丹术为代表的道家气功重视体内精气神的作用，并强调心神的主导地位，提出了著名的三炼，即炼精化气、炼气化神及炼神还虚，最后合于大道而得长生。

Taoism has a long history in Chinese culture. Historically, Taoist qigong can be traced far back to Lao Zi and Zhuang Zi in the pre-Qin period (BCE 770–BCE 221). Following the Han Dynasty, Taoism integrated the thoughts and techniques of other schools, including health cultivation, yin-yang theory, medicine, and witchcraft. It also merged Taoist theories with the practice of Taoist practitioners. Taoist qigong thereafter underwent further development. This exercise is characterized by cultivation of both body and mind and represented by internal alchemy, also known as Zhou Tian Gong (Heavenly Circle Qigong). The internal alchemy focuses on the internal exercise of essence, qi and spirit and proposes three refining — refining essence into qi, refining qi into spirit and refining spirit into emptiness, eventually achieving Dao.

道家气功主要指道家成仙之学中的一些修炼技术，修炼注重养生长寿，其提倡的修炼技术实用且易于操作，例如导引吐纳、抱一守中、炼丹服食、胎息辟谷、性命双修等。从气功学角度看，道家气功始于老庄，练功的一些基本原则如"道法自然""虚静无为""返朴归真"等，在老庄的著作中已经奠定，故《老子》《庄子》不仅在中国哲学史上名列鳌头，在中国气功史上也占有极其重要地位。

Taoist qigong mainly refers to cultivation techniques in the Taoist immortal theory, which focuses on nourishing health and achieving longevity. It advocates exercises that are easy to practice, such as Tu Na (breathing in and breathing out) and Daoyin, Bao Yi Shou Zhong (embraces the One and cultivates *Yuan*-primordial qi), ingestion of immortality pills, fetal (embryonic) breathing, Bi Gu (fasting) and dual cultivation of inherent nature and life endowment. From the qigong perspective, Daoist qigong starts from the philosophy of Zhuang Zi, such as "following Dao", "inaction", and "returning to one's original purity". In this sense, the *Laozi* and *Zhuangzi* are not only influential in philosophy but also in the history of qigong.

逍遥行步功是道家逍遥功的一部分，与逍遥动功一起都属于古传道家导引术，《庄子》中曾这样描写："吐故纳新，熊经鸟伸，为寿而已矣。"这其中的"熊经鸟伸"，就是对古代养生之士模仿动物姿势习练气功的描述。逍遥行步功是由上海市气功研究所董妙成医师所传行步功法之一。这是一种很特别的练功方法，通过把肢体导引、站桩桩功和静心冥想相结合，使三调合一，进入一种恍惚杳冥的深层练功态，日久功深，能使腿脚轻健有力，体内真气充足，心神宁静祥和，并起到养生健身、调理脏腑、祛病康复的功用。

As one part of Xiao Yao Gong (Free and Easy Exercise), Xiao Yao qigong exercise in walking falls under the category of Taoist Daoyin exercise. The *Zhuangzi* states, "exhale the old and inhale the new, walk like a bear and stretch the neck like a bird to achieve longevity". The "walking like a bear and stretching like a bird" is a vivid description of ancient health people imitating animal postures and movements. *Xiao Yao* qigong exercise in walking was inherited and taught by qigong master Dong Miaocheng in Shanghai Qigong Research Institute. This special qigong method aims to strengthen the body, supplement the genuine qi and tranquilize the mind through Daoyin, post standing exercise and meditation, eventually achieving the unity of the three regulations to cultivate health, regulate zang-fu organs and recover from diseases.

逍遥行步功手的姿势（图2-1）与脚的姿势（图2-2）。

The position of the hands (Figure 2–1) and feet (Figure 2–2).

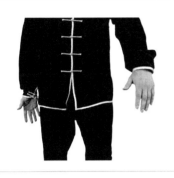

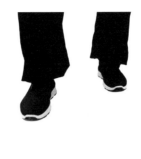

图2-1　Figure 2–1　　　　图2-2　Figure 2–2

预备式
Preparation Movement

两脚略分开，间距可容纳下并排两拳为宜，自然站立，全身放松，两眼平视前方，收视返听，略微调理呼吸，宁心安神。（图2-3、图2-4）

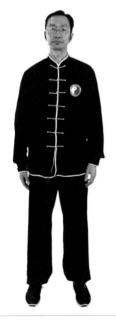

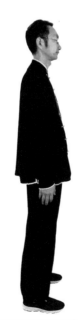

图2-3　Figure 2–3　　　　图2-4　Figure 2–4

Separate the feet to shoulder-width apart. Stand naturally with a relaxed body and refreshed mind. Look straight ahead, regulate breathing and tranquilize the mind. (Figure 2–3 and Figure 2–4)

操作要领
Tips

1. 调身
1. Body Regulation

两腿缓缓屈膝下坐（图2-5），起步时重心移向右腿，坐实右腿并保持稳定，轻轻提起左腿，左脚略上提向前迈步，距离为一个脚掌，同时重心保持在右腿，身体略转胯向左并带动右手往前撩，掌心向前（图2-6）。接着略向右转胯，带动左手转掌心往前撩，同时右手转掌往后（图2-7）。接着再次转胯向左，同时右手前撩左手往回带（图2-8）。

Slowly bend the knees to lower the body (Figure 2–5). Place the body weight on the right leg and slowly stand up while maintaining stability. Slightly lift the left leg and step forward with the left foot at one-foot length. Keep the body weight on the right leg, slightly turn the hip to the left, and stretch the right hand with the palm forward (Figure 2–6). Then slightly turn the hip to the right, stretch the left hand with the palm facing forward, and move the right hand backward (Figure 2–7). After that, turn the hip to the left again, stretch the right hand with the palm forward, and move the left hand backward (Figure 2–8).

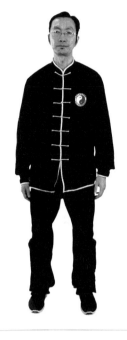

图2-5　Figure 2-5

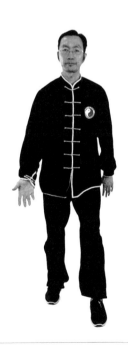

图2-6　Figure 2-6

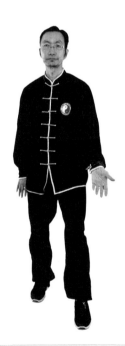

图2-7　Figure 2-7

图2-8　Figure 2-8

重心逐渐前移，慢慢坐稳左腿，轻轻提起右腿，左脚略上提向前迈步，距离为一个脚掌，同时身体略转胯向右并带动左手往前撩，掌心向前。以下动作姿势相同，唯方向相反。（图2-9～图2-11）

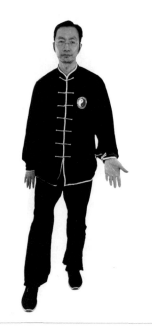 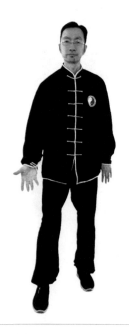

图2-9　Figure 2-9　　　　　图2-10　Figure 2-10

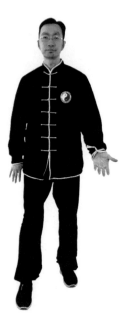

图2-11　Figure 2-11

Move the body weight forward to the left leg, slightly lift the right leg, and move the left foot one step forward. Meanwhile, slightly turn the hip to the right and stretch the left hand with the palm forward. Repeat the movements in the same posture but in the opposite direction. (Figure 2-9 to Figure 2-11)

直线向前行步,速度以缓慢为宜,越慢越好,行至尽头收势右脚并左脚同时站直,转身分脚站立,再开步往回行步。

Move forward for a few steps as slow as possible, retract the right foot, and place the feet together to stand upright, then turn around, separate the feet, and repeat the above walking movements.

2. 调息
2. Breath Regulation

在做行步功时保持柔和自然的呼吸,以后呼吸渐渐细微。

Maintain soft and natural breathing while practicing qigong exercise in walking, and then your breathing will gradually become slower and slower.

3. 调心
3. Mind Regulation

初练之时使心神专注于动作姿势的正确,熟练后如在水中前行,两手摆动如划水前行。并且慢慢可体会人在气中、气在人中的感受。

It's advisable for beginners to concentrate their minds on the posture and movements. After some time, one can gradually feel like walking forward in the water with two hands swinging like paddles. Moreover, one can start to experience the unity of qi and body.

注意事项
Notes

（1）在做行功时要保持上身正直平稳，上身不能摇晃，在转胯时重心不能移动，要坐实后腿。

(1) When walking, keep the upper body upright and stable, do not move the body weight when turning the hips, while the back leg should remain stable.

（2）练习时以高位姿势为主，两膝不超过脚尖为宜，但要循序渐进，逐渐增加习练时间，以达到日久功深的目的。

(2) Keep the high position with the knees slightly bent when practicing, but do not let the knees go past the toes. Gradually, one can increase the exercise time to make progress.

（3）身体转胯是主动，带动上身、两臂及两掌摆动，同时两臂摆动要圆活自然。

(3) Turning the hip may move the upper body, arms and palms together. Swing the arms naturally.

应用
Application

本功法以慢步行功为主要形式，把肢体导引、站桩桩功和静心冥想相结合，通过习练可以进入三调合一的较深的气功境界，达到形气神相合奇妙状态，对许多慢性病如高血压、失眠、支气管炎、胃肠炎等较好的调理作用。

This exercise uses slow walking as the main form and combines Daoyin, post standing exercise and meditation. Through practice, one can step into the advanced stage of qigong, that is, the unity of the three regulations (regulating the body, breath and mind).This exercise is helpful to chronic diseases including hypertension, insomnia, bronchitis and gastrointestinal disorders.

三、佛家行禅法
Walking Meditation in Buddhism

佛教是于东汉初年开始由印度传入的，魏晋南北朝时得到较快发展，至隋唐达到鼎盛。佛教讲究修持，如从增进、深化身心健康的角度解读其修持，便可将其中有关心身、呼吸操作的内容归为气功修炼，这便是佛家气功产生的背景。从气功特色看，佛家气功以调心为主，注重调心与调息的结合。其功法以静为多，代表功法是"禅定"。

Buddhism was introduced from India in the early years of the Eastern Han Dynasty and well developed during the Wei, Jin, Southern and Northern Dynasties (266–589), reaching its peak in the Sui and Tang Dynasties (281–907). Buddhism focuses on cultivation. If we understand it from the perspective of enhancing and strengthening physical and mental health, the content regarding mind, body and breathing can be categorized into qigong practice. This is the origin of Buddhism qigong. In terms of qigong, Buddhism qigong focuses on mind regulation and highlights the combination of mind regulation and breathing regulation. It is mostly static and represented by meditation.

佛家气功主要指佛家修持的禅定、止观等方法和技术，佛家的修持注重戒、定、慧三学。戒学是戒律的修习，指趋善去恶等道德修养，以坚强的信念来控制自己的心理和行为。定学是禅定的修习，气功中也叫入定。禅定包括"止""观"两个方面，"止"是以一念代万念，逐渐减少杂念和思维活动，以达到心如明镜止水。"观"是在定的状态下洞察心灵，以获得净化和解脱。慧学是智慧的修习，在修定的基础上想要获得超越性的大智慧。佛家通过戒、定、慧三学进行修炼，以达成修身养性的最高境界。

Buddhism qigong refers to the methods and techniques practiced by Buddhists, such as concentrated meditation and insight meditation. Commandment, contemplation and wisdom are the essences of Buddhism. Commandment refers to moral cultivation as well as control of one's mind and behavior through strong beliefs. Contemplation is the practice of meditation and has two parts, namely, mind concentration and insightful observation. The mind concentration can help to remove distracting thoughts, replace the ten thousand thoughts with one singe thought and gradually become meditative. The insightful observation can acquire mental purification and relief. Wisdom refers to the outstanding wisdom through learning.

佛家行禅法又名经行。经行是佛家禅修者在静坐之后，来回地直线地专注地行走。经行是一个人单独完成，经行在初学者，仍然是修定的一种，直到有了定力之后，也可以变成修观，因为修定是一个比较漫长的过程。

After seated meditation, those who practice Buddhist meditation can walk back and forth in a straight line with mental focus. This is called walking meditation. Walking meditation is done by one person alone and it may take time and efforts to cultivate contemplation of mind for beginners.

佛家禅修者，很多人不能坚持下去，是因为没有真正得到禅定的好处，而没有禅悦作支撑，这条路就很难走下去。很多初学者很大的毛病，就是修定的时间少，然后行禅、经行的时间几乎没有。如果没有尝到禅修的好处，打坐就成了一种痛苦，因为不知道如何动静用功。他们不能坚持下去有两方面原因，内因来说他的道心不够，厌离心不够，所以他浅尝辄止，遇到困难就选择了放弃。从技术层面来说，是投入时间少，投入方式是动静结合不够，就像登山一样，如不适当地使用体力，就会把自己弄得太疲劳、太痛苦。

As they don't actually experience the benefits of meditation, many people give up the path. It is challenging for beginners to stick to the path without the support of meditation pleasure. Many beginners devote little time to practicing meditation and even less time to walking. Therefore, they find meditation painful since they don't know how to walk and make use of their energy. They can't keep on for two reasons. First, they haven't developed a pure mind free of distracting thoughts, and therefore they tend to give up when things get tough. Second, they need to spend more time on technique and learn to combine movement and stillness during exercise. This is like mountain climbing. Improper use of physical strength will make one exhausted and uncomfortable.

静坐之后，可用经行、行禅来作辅助禅修，而不是静坐之后马上忙于工作，要把时间安排好，不能只有静坐时间，没有经行时间。初学者的经行只要注意自己呼吸就好，或者注意自己的行动都可以，觉知行动是第一选择，就是你抬起脚，然后向前，然后落下，然后接触，然后感知接触地面的感觉，然后来回地缓慢走。行禅会发展觉知的平衡性、准确性与专注的持久性，在行禅时可观察到很深奥的佛法，甚至获得证悟。因此佛家禅修者多在打坐之余行经行之事。

For beginners, the time should be properly arranged. Instead of jumping into work right away after seated meditation, walking meditation may serve as a useful technique. Keep slow walking, concentrating attention on the breathing or movements, such as the feet raising, stepping, and touching the ground. Walking meditation helps to improve balance, accuracy and persistence of awareness and concentration. During walking, one may have an epiphany. Therefore, in addition to sitting, Buddhists also practice meditation walking.

操作要领
Tips

经行的操作分为快速经行和慢速经行两类，要求将心系在走路的感觉上。

Walking meditation can be fast or slow, both of which require mental focus when walking.

1. 快步经行

1. Fast-speed Walking Meditation

（1）预备式：松静站立，两足略开立；双膝双胯自然放松，身体重心落于两足中间。双臂自然下垂，手指自然微弯曲；沉肩坠肘，虚腋松腕，含胸拔背，百会朝天，松腰敛臀。两目先平视远方，舌抵上腭，神态自然。（图3-1）

（1）Preparation posture: Stand in relaxation and tranquility with separated feet, relax the knees and hips, and put the body weight in the middle of the two feet. Drop the arms naturally to the sides with slightly flexed fingers. Sink the shoulders and drop the elbows, relax the upper limbs and armpits, tuck the chest in and pull up the back, relax the waist, tuck the buttocks and keep the head upright. Look straight ahead and touch the palate with the tongue with a natural facial expression. (Figure 3-1)

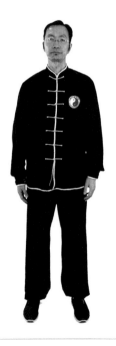

图3-1　Figure 3-1

（2）调身：习练者注意走路的每个步骤，以较快的速度向前走去，保持身体松静自然中正，两臂自然摆动，注意腿部的移动，心中默念"左、右、左、右"，并觉知整个腿部的实际感觉。（图3-2～图3-5）

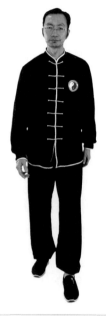

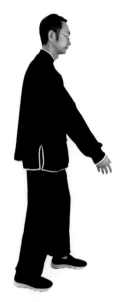

图3-2　Figure 3-2　　　　　　　　图3-3　Figure 3-3

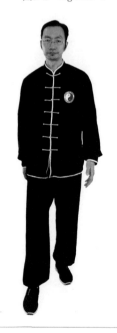

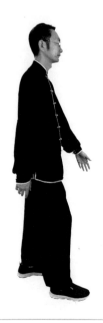

图3-4　Figure 3-4　　　　　　　　图3-5　Figure 3-5

(2) Body regulation: Focus on each stride of the walk, move forward at a faster speed, keep a relaxed, upright posture, and swing both arms naturally. Pay attention to the movements of the legs. While being conscious of the entire leg, chant silently in the head, "Left, right, left, right." (Figure 3–2 to Figure 3–5)

2. 慢步经行
2. Slow-speed Walking Meditation

（1）预备式：松静站立，两足略开立，双膝双胯自然放松，身体重心落于两足中间。两手背于身后，沉肩坠肘，虚腋松腕，含胸拔背，百会朝天。松腰敛臀，两目先平视远方，舌抵上腭，神态自然。

(1) Preparation posture: Stand in relaxation and tranquility with separated feet, relax the knees and hips, and put the body weight in the middle of the two feet. Put both hands behind the back. Sink the shoulders and drop the elbows, relax the upper limbs and armpits, tuck the chest in and pull up the back, relax the waist, tuck the buttocks and keep the head upright. Look straight ahead and touch the palate with the tongue with a natural facial expression.

（2）调身：习练者以固定的、庄重的、优雅的姿势，将两手背于身后，保持这个固定的姿势，迈步向前走出，自己的整个身心不仅要正直，还要放松，保持舒适、喜悦的心、宁静的心，来回地慢慢地走，每一步就是一脚掌半，全脚掌着地，经行的长度是十米到十五米之间，不能少于十米，不能超过十五米，在尽头处缓慢地有觉知的转身，然后继续这样专注地慢慢地走。（图3-6～图3-9）

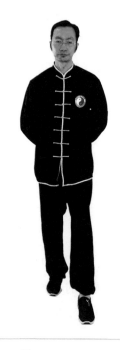

图3-6　Figure 3-6

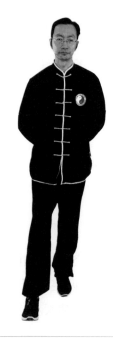

图3-7　Figure 3-7

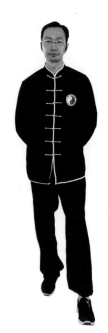

图3-8　Figure 3-8

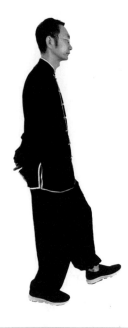

图3-9　Figure 3-9

(2) Body regulation: Keep the body relaxed and upright while moving ahead with a dignified and graceful posture. Place both hands behind the back. Walk back and forth slowly, make strides that are each one and a half feet in length, and step fully onto the ground. Move forward for about ten to fifteen meters, turn around slowly at the end, and then continue walking slowly with this concentration. (Figure 3-6 to Figure 3-9)

（3）调息：保持自然呼吸，并渐渐达到忘息。

(3) Breath regulation: Keep breathing naturally and gradually reach fetal breathing (embryonic respiration).

（4）调心：习练经行时要专心觉知腿脚运动过程中的感觉。

(4) Mind regulation: Concentrate on the sensations of the legs and feet during the movement.

注意事项
Notes

经行时间、行禅时间不低于静坐时间的30%，应该在30%～50%之间。初学者每天静坐2次，每坐不少于30分钟，然后应该经行、行禅1～2次或更多。要注意每一脚的抬起、移动与放下，不论任何一种情况，都要努力的完全把心系在走路的感觉上。当你走到步道尽头，立定、转身再度开步时，都要注意有什么动作发生。除非遇到地上有障碍物，否则不要低头看脚，当致力于觉知感觉时，你要专注于感觉本身，而不是视觉的影像。通常将行禅分成三个不同的动作——将脚抬起、移动、放下。为了维持精确的觉知，需要清楚地区分这些动作，在开始时，心中轻轻地默念每个动作，并让觉知确实清楚、有力地跟随，直到动作结束。初学者20～40分钟都可以，结束之后可以放松身心。注意经行的时间是在静坐之后，饭后不宜经行，如果饭后经行，需要等30分钟，因为它的专注会影响胃部的消化。

Walking meditation time should be no less than 30% of the seated meditation and should be between 30% and 50%. Beginners may practice seated meditation twice a day for no less than 30 minutes each time, and then practice walking meditation once or twice or more. Focus on the lifting, moving, and placing down of each foot. In any case, concentrate on the feeling of walking instead of the visual image. When you reach the end of the step, stand still, turn around and start walking again. Don't look down at your feet unless you encounter an obstacle. Lifting the feet up, moving them, and putting them down are three distinct steps of walking meditation. It is essential to differentiate between these movements in order to retain precise awareness. Begin by focusing the attention on each mental activity, allowing your awareness to track it vividly and intently all the way through. It's advisable for beginners to practice walking meditation for 20–40 minutes each time. After the practice, one can relax the body and mind. It's worth noting that walking meditation should be practiced after seated meditation or at least 30 minutes after eating food, because the concentration may affect the digestion.

应用
Application

（1）常练习行禅的人，可以增强长途旅行的耐力，这在佛陀时代特别重要，当时的比丘与比丘尼，除了双脚以外，没有其他交通工具。

(1) Practicing walking meditation regularly may increase your stamina for long trip. It was vital in the time of the Buddha, when Buddhist monks and nuns had no other means of transportation than their feet.

（2）增加禅修本身的耐力。行禅需要双倍的精进，除了用来抬脚的一般机械性的精进之外，还需要心的精进来觉知动作——这正是八正道中的正精进。如果这种双倍的精进持续在整个抬脚、向前与放下的动作中，能强化有力而稳定的心的精进能量，这对修观十分重要。

(2) It can enhance the stamina of the meditation. In addition to the movement of lifting and placing down the feet, the practitioner also needs to concentrate on the walking itself. As part of the right effort of the Ba Zheng Dao (the Noble Eightfold Path) in Buddhism, walking meditation requires double efforts. If the double efforts continue throughout the lifting, stepping forwards, and placing down the feet, it strengthens mental energy, which is very important for the contemplation of mind.

（3）坐禅与行禅之间的平衡有益健康，两者交替，会使禅修的进步速度加快。生病时很难禅修，坐太久会导致许多身体失调的状况，但交换姿势与行禅的动作，会使肌肉复苏，促进血液循环与预防疾病。

(3) The balance between seated meditation and walking meditation is beneficial to health. Alternating between the two may result in faster progress in meditation. It is difficult to practice meditation when you are ill, since sitting for too long may cause physical disorders, but switching between sitting

and walking can relax the muscles, improve blood circulation and prevent illness.

（4）帮助消化。消化不良会导致很多不舒服的感觉，因而成为修习的障碍。行禅能促进肠胃蠕动，保持通畅。饭后与禅坐前应该要进行一段行禅，以驱逐睡意。

(4) Walking meditation helps digestion. Poor digestion may cause uncomfortable sensations and thus become an obstacle to practice. Walking meditation can promote bowel movements. Therefore, it should be practiced after a meal and before seated meditation to prevent drowsiness.

（5）建立持久的专注。由于心在行走时集中于动作的每个部分，专注便会持续不断。每个脚步都在为接下来的禅坐建立基础。

(5) Cultivate lasting concentration. Concentration continues when you walk as the mind concentrates on each step of the movement. Each step lays the groundwork for the seated meditation.

四、郭林新气功
Guo Lin Qigong

郭林新气功是由郭林女士整理创编的一种新型气功，由传统的儒家、道家、佛家、医家、武术等的功理功法中，去粗取精，集各家所长，推陈出新，逐渐形成了自己的医疗功法体系，属于医家气功的范畴。新气功疗法是在吸收华佗五禽戏长处的基础上创编，以"行功"为主要练功方式的功法。它将传统气功中的意念导引、呼吸导引、形体导引有机地结合起来，同时又将意念导引作为整套功法核心，使动静相兼，动中求静，静中有动。新气功疗法在调息上的独特之处是采用"风呼吸法"，呼吸快、猛、强。此法在清晨习练，可吸收大量的氧气，故利于产生较强的内气。

Guo Lin qigong was a type of qigong therapy developed by Ms. Guo Lin. It incorporates the essence of traditional Confucianism, Taoism, Buddhism, TCM, and martial arts and falls under the category of medical qigong. The new qigong therapy was based on Hua Tuo's Wu Qin Xi, using walking as the main form of exercise. Guo Lin qigong combines motion and stillness, including intent Daoyin, breathing Daoyin and body Daoyin of traditional qigong, highlighting the intent Daoyin. Its distinctive function is to regulate breathing with quick, forceful and strong, which is known as "wind breathing." By practicing this in the morning, one can inhale abundant oxygen to generate internal qi.

郭林新气功分为三个层次，初级功，中级功，高级功；分五个导引，意念导引，呼吸导引，势子导引，吐音导引，综合按摩导引。其中以慢步行功、升降开合、三关分渡为总的功法核心。

Guo Lin qigong consists of three stages — primary, intermediate, and advanced — and five Daoyin techniques: intent Daoyin, breathing Daoyin, body Daoyin, sound Daoyin, and Tuina Daoyin. Among them, the slow qigong exercise in walking, ascending, descending, opening and closing, and three regulations are especially important.

人为什么会生病？一般来说，"患生于多欲而人心难测""傲不可长，欲不可纵，志不可满，乐不可极"。大多先由七情六欲不知节制，百忧感心，万事劳形，使身心、阴阳、脏腑、经络、气血常规失调，破坏功能平衡所致。人若练功，可使身心、阴阳、经络、气血运行畅通，恢复平衡，病自痊愈。

Why do people become sick? "The root cause is greed and desire." As the saying goes, "Pride, desire, will and joy should not be excessive". The imbalance of the seven emotions and six sensory pleasures may affect yin, yang, zang-fu organs, meridians, qi and blood. Practicing qigong can restore yin-yang balance, benefit the body and mind, and promote the circulation of qi and blood.

五种导引以意念导引为全功主导，意念活动包括思想、感情、意识、思维等活动。人的言动行止，时时处处都必先由意识发动（有意无意），所谓万事成败在于一念之动能否坚持贯彻始终。练功也是如此，常说"全凭心意用功夫""大道教人先止念，念头不止也枉然"。人自无始有生以来，即有杂念不断生起，要练意念就是使精神高度集中，达到静定境界（似入无念境，其实尚有微细念头）。新气功意念导引功法中，把意念活动集中到某一点、某一词或某一事物上，借以排除各种纷纭的杂念，即所谓"以一念代万念""制心一处无事不办"。通过这种功法使大脑皮层逐渐进入并长时间保持在既不兴奋又不抑制的入静状态（无住生心，定慧平等，寂而常照的气功态）。

The intent Daoyin plays a pivotal role in qigong exercise. Mental activities include thoughts, feelings, consciousness, and thinking. A person's words, actions and behaviors must be initiated by mental processes (intentionally or unintentionally). The same is true for qigong practice. It is often said that "Kung fu is all about the mental intention" and "to pursue Dao, one must learn how to remove distracting thoughts." Since the beginning of our lives, wandering thoughts have existed in everyone's mind. The aim of intent Daoyin is to focus the mind and achieve a state of tranquility (it seems to be in the state of no-thought, but there are still subtle thoughts). It's advisable to focus the mind on a word or object to eliminate all distracting thoughts. This is known as "replacing ten thousand thoughts with one thought" and "focusing the mind on one." Through this exercise, the cerebral cortex can gradually enter and remain a state of tranquility that is neither excited nor inhibited for a long time (a deep meditative state of mind or a qigong state of mindfulness, serenity and tranquility without distracting thoughts).

呼吸引导是佛家天台宗止观法门的下手处,在《小止观》和《六妙门》中讲得具体明确。所谓"调息",要求把呼吸练到深匀细长。呼吸有风、喘、气、息四种不同的状态,前三者为不调之相,后者为调相。而郭林新气功为治疗癌症、重症,特别改革为短促的风呼吸。然而风呼吸是被古人认为练功禁忌的。

Breathing Daoyin is the key to practice contemplation in Tiantai Sect, which has been clearly explained in *Xiao Zhi Guan* (Introduction to Contemplation) and *Liu Miao Men* (The Six Entrances of Enlightenment). Breathing regulation aims to reach "deep, even, long and soft" breathing. There are four phases of breathing: unhurried breathing (*feng*), panting (*chuan*), deep and quiet breathing (*qi*) and stillness or rest (*xi*). The first three types of breathing are incorrect, while the fourth is correct. To deal with diseases, Guo Lin qigong changed the unhurried breathing into fast and short, which is contraindicated in qigong practice by ancient people.

吐音导引是郭林新气功特有的功法之一。它根据《黄帝内经》藏象学说,人体五脏有五音,肝角、心徵、脾宫、肺商、肾羽。

吐音功法约言三句话：三松、三稳、丹田气。天地间最微妙的事物是声音，转瞬即逝；最大的威力是雷电，春雷一震万物复苏。人患疾病，五脏失调，各种功能常规紊乱，辨证吐音可相应引起五脏功能共振同鸣，使之恢复常态，所以可祛病。

Sound Daoyin is a unique therapy of Guo Lin qigong. According to the Zangxiang theory in *Huang Di Nei Jing*, the five organs of the human body correspond to five notes: *Jiao* (liver), *Zhi* (heart), *Gong* (spleen), *Shang* (lung), and *Yu* (kidney). Sound Daoyin can be summed up in three parts: relaxation, stability, and qi of Dantian. The most subtle thing in heaven and earth is sound, because it is ephemeral. The greatest power is thunder and lightning, just as the spring thunder awakens all lives. Dysfunctions of the five-zang organs may cause diseases. Practicing sound Daoyin can resonate with the five-zang organs and help to restore their normal functions and eliminate diseases.

势子导引多是据华佗五禽戏及易筋经、武术、太极、八卦等创编的。

Body Daoyin is developed on the basis of Wu Qin Xi, Yi Jin Jing (Sinew-Transformation Classic), martial arts, Taiji and Ba Gua (Eight-Diagram).

慢步行功是郭林新气功特殊的步法。这种步法功理在一动一静行止之间，具备了五禽戏的形神兼备的姿态，看起来似乎很简单、容易学，其实要认真学好是不容易的。太极拳、八卦掌即是这种步法，所谓"迈步如猫行、运劲若抽丝"。一脚跟先着地落实后，再换另一脚，两足虚实分明，头部左顾右盼，可以调理肾与膀胱经气血运行。

Slow walking is a unique footwork used in Guo Lin qigong. It combines motion with stillness, manifesting the feature of Wu Qin Xi. Although it seems simple to learn, it's not easy to learn it well. Taijiquan and Ba Gua Palm also include slow walking, which is often described as "stepping like a cat walking and exerting force like drawing silk". During exercise, one should first land on one heel, then switch to the other foot while turning the head to the left and right. In this way, the qi and blood of kidney and bladder meridians can be regulated.

郭林新气功典型功法之一是"三关分渡"。把三者分开，先练松静，次练调息，后练意守，讲究掌握意、气、形。意指意念活动；气是内气；形是形体动作，即是势子。练功就要练出内气，要想更多地产生内气，就要正确使用各种导引法，过好三关（即松静关、调息关、意念关），其中意念活动起关键作用。意、气、形三字，古人以形神二字概括。

One of the unique techniques in Guo Lin qigong is called "three separated passes," namely, relaxation, breathing and mental focus. Practice body relaxation first, then breathing regulation, then mental concentration. The intent, qi and posture are essential in the whole process. The intent refers to consciousness; qi means internal qi; posture means body movements. To overcome the three passes (relaxation, breathing and mental focus), one needs to use Daoyin methods, especially the mental focus.

郭林新气功的任何功法，都要做到圆、软、远。圆是在练功时，躯干身体各节保持圆形，各关节不要僵直，这是依据太极圆周运行不息而来的。软是通过练功使身体肢节松软，不要僵硬死板，"松而不懈""柔中有刚"是本源。远是闭眼练功时平视前方，不可上视、下视或斜视。初练功时，意念应集中在体外。若认真做到此三字诀，才能更多地产生内气。

Round, soft, and far are characteristics of Guo Lin qigong. The "round" means flexible movements without causing joint rigidity. The "soft" means soft limbs and flexible joints. The "far" means looking forward during practice. For beginners, it's advisable to place the mental focus on the outside of the body. Only by this way, can one generate more internal qi.

综上所述，新气功疗法内容较多，包括定步风呼吸、升降开合慢步行功、快步行功、中度风呼吸自然行功，中度风呼吸一、二、三步行功，以及吐音导引和各种复式按摩等功法。临床上常用中度风呼吸法自然行功防治疾病，用中度风呼吸法一、二、三步行功辅助防癌抗癌，本节仅介绍中度风呼吸法自然行功。

In conclusion, Guo Lin qigong includes fixed-step wind breathing, slow qigong exercise in walking, fast qigong exercise in walking, natural qigong exercise in walking with moderate-speed wind breathing, qigong exercise in walking with moderate-speed wind breathing (one, two or three steps), sound Daoyin and compound massage techniques. In clinical settings, qigong exercise in walking with moderate-speed wind-breathing is often used to prevent and treat diseases, and qigong exercise in walking with moderate-speed wind-breathing (one, two or three steps) is often used to prevent cancer. In this chapter, we will introduce natural qigong exercise in walking with moderate-speed wind-breathing.

所谓中度风呼吸法就是指行走的速度是中等的，呼吸的速度也是中等的。这种中度风呼吸法比较平稳，适应多种慢性疾病及癌症患者，除严重的心脏病外一般均可应用。本功法强调"松静自然"，因此从外形上看好似闲庭信步。其操作要领强调"圆、软、远"三字诀。圆，是指练功时躯干和肢体动作要保持圆或弧线形的运动姿态，要神情自然，动作圆满，气势一贯；软，是指运动时肩、头、颈、躯干、臀、腿、腰等部位要保持一定的松软，不要僵硬死板；远，是指眼睛无论是半闭半合或是轻轻闭合，都要向前平观远方，要做到视而不见，见而不盯，切不可低头看地。练功过程中若能以此三字诀对照检查，效果才明显。

With moderate walking and breathing, this qigong exercise is suitable for patients with chronic diseases or cancer but not suitable for those with severe heart disease. Natural qigong exercise in walking with moderate-speed wind-breathing appears to be a leisurely stroll because it is relaxed, soft and even with constant speed and mind-qi unity. The practice emphasizes the three words "round, soft and far." The "round" describes round movements of the torso and limbs. The "soft" shows up as relaxed shoulders, head, neck, torso, buttocks, legs and waist. The "far" refers to the far-looking gaze, either closed or half-open.

中度风呼吸法自然行功
Natural Qigong Exercise in Walking with Moderate-speed Wind-breathing

操作要领
Tips

1. 调身
1. Body Regulation

（1）预备功：松静站立，两足平行开立，与肩同宽，两膝微曲，不超过足尖，双膝双胯自然放松，身体重心落于两足中间。

双臂自然下垂,置于两腿的外侧稍前方,手指自然微弯曲,沉肩坠肘,虚腋松腕,含胸拔背,百会朝天。松腰、收腹、沉胯。两目先平视远方片刻,然后再缓慢轻轻地闭合,舌抵上腭,神态自然。(图4-1)

(1) Preparation posture: Separate the legs to stand naturally and comfortably. Parallel the feet to shoulder-width apart, slightly bend the knees but do not let the knees go past the toes and put the body weight in the middle of the feet. Drop the arms naturally to the sides with slightly flexed fingers. Sink the shoulders and drop the elbows, relax the upper limbs and armpits, tuck the chest in and pull up the back, relax the waist, tuck in the belly, relax the hip joints and keep the head upright. Look straight ahead for a while, and then slowly close the eyes. Touch the palate with the tongue with a natural facial expression. (Figure 4-1)

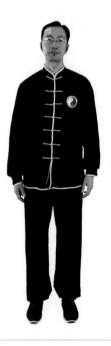

图4-1　Figure 4-1

松静站立是新气功疗法各种行功的一个基础势子，通过此势能使心安神静，气血流通，所以要严格按照练功的具体要领操作，不可草率行事。

Beginners shall strictly adhere to the movements, since it is a basic posture for tranquilizing the mind and circulating qi and blood.

中丹田三个气呼吸：气呼吸即是鼻吸口呼的呼吸。松静站立后，双手轻缓地由胯旁向中丹田聚拢，开始时两手心相对，指尖向下，待移至中丹田时两掌心转向腹部，先将左手（男先左、女先右）的劳宫穴贴于肚脐处，再将右手（女为左手）掌心重叠在左手手背，使左右手的内、外劳宫穴相叠。双手位置放好后，开始做呼吸动作。先用口呼，随呼气两腿慢慢下蹲，使身体缓慢下降；呼气尽时身体不动，用鼻吸气，先呼后吸为补，体虚久病者较为适宜。当吸气满后稍憋住，待身体上升，两腿慢慢直立后再呼气。整个呼吸过程为一呼、一吸、一平，为一个气呼吸，共做3次。（图4-2）

Qi breathing patterns of the middle Dantian: Qi breathing is nose-in and mouth-out breathing. After the standing posture, extend the hands to the middle Dantian with the palms facing each other and fingertips downward. Then, move the hand to the abdomen, cover the umbilicus with Laogong (PC8) of the left hand (man with left hand first and woman with right hand first), then place the right hand on the left hand, with overlapped Laogong (PC8) of both hands on the umbilicus. After this, the breathing practice shall begin. First, exhale with the mouth while slowly squatting and lowering the body. After the expiration, keep the body still and inhale with the nose. Then, hold the breath for a while, slowly stand up, and exhale with the mouth after both legs stand upright. The whole process of qi breathing consists of three parts: exhalation, inhalation, and

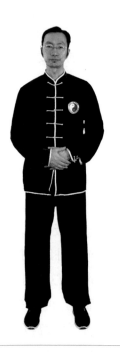

图4-2　Figure 4-2

pause. Repeat three times. (Figure 4–2)

［注意事项］三个气呼吸要遵循自然的原则，切不可用力或勉强追求深长，不可用力呼尽吸足。用口呼气时，口不要张得太大，微露一缝即可；要松腰、松胯、松膝，身体随着呼气作缓慢的下降。下降的位置和降速可根据自己的病情而定。如高血压病人，身体下降的位置可以低一些，速度慢一点，而低血压不做下蹲动作。呼到一定程度后，就开始吸气，吸时身体先不要伴随上升动作，保持呼气时的原位，切不要边吸边直立身体，以免胸部发生不适感或憋气现象，一定要吸完后再慢慢地直立起来。

[Notes] The qi breathing pattern requires natural breathing. Remember to avoid exhaling or inhaling excessively while practicing. When inhaling, keep the mouth partly open; relax the knees, hips, and waist; and lower the body slowly as you exhale. The position and speed can be adjusted according to individual conditions. For example, people with high blood pressure should lower the body slowly and people with low blood pressure do not lower the body. When exhaling to a certain point, keep your body still, slowly stand up, and then inhale to prevent chest discomfort.

通过三个气呼吸，促使大脑逐渐进入轻松可控制的安静状态，使失调的大脑功能得到合理的调整，充分地恢复大脑的功能。

Three qi breathing can help the brain enter a relaxed and controllable tranquil state and thus fully restore the brain functions.

中丹田三开合：① 开法：最后一个呼吸结束后，恢复自然呼吸。然后将双手从"抱丹田"式向体两侧慢慢地分开。开时两手手背相对，掌心向外，手指并拢。开到略比自己的身体稍宽些为止，此称为一"开"。② 合法：开后，双手同时缓慢翻掌，变掌心相对，并向腹前丹田处聚拢至双手将要接触而尚未接触时止，称为一"合"。一开一合反复做三次，称中丹田三开合。（图4-3、图4-4）

Opening and closing of the middle Dantian: ① Opening method: After practicing qi breathing of the middle Dantian, restore natural breathing. Then open and separate the hands to the sides with the dorsum of the hand facing each other. ② Closing method: After the opening, slowly turn over the palms and make two palms facing each other, then move the palms to cover the Dantian over the abdomen without touching. Repeat three times and complete three openings and closings of the middle Dantian. (Figure 4-3 and Figure 4-4)

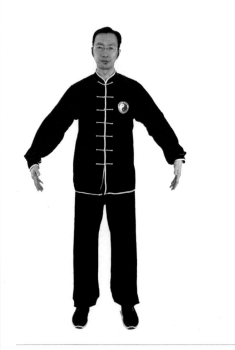

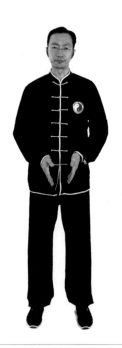

图4-3　Figure 4-3　　　　　　图4-4　Figure 4-4

［注意事项］丹田开合时要意守丹田。意守丹田可以生发元气，调和血脉，增强脾胃功能。

[Notes] Keep the mental focus on the Dantian to activate *Yuan*-primordial qi, harmonize blood and vessels and strengthen the spleen and stomach.

（2）行功：迈步法。预备功后，慢慢睁开双目，目光平视前方，然后像散步似地向前行走。行功出脚的顺序一般依照男左女右的原则（即男子先迈左腿，女子先迈右腿），若是病患者，可根据不同的病症决定出脚的次序。如高血压、心脏病患者，可以不分男女，一律先左后右。肝病患者与之相反，先右后左；癌症患者根据病情所在一侧，决定出脚次序。以先迈左脚为例，左腿迈出，左脚跟先轻轻着地，前脚掌自然竖起，随身体重心的左移，左脚自然放平，再开始迈右脚，变右脚脚跟先着地，脚掌自然竖起，随身体的重心右移，右脚逐渐放平。如此左右交替，一步一步地向前走。（图4-5～图4-7）

(2) Walking: Stepping method. After preparation, slowly open the eyes, look straight ahead, and walk forward just like you're going for a stroll. Men should step with their left foot first, and women should step with their right foot first. People with hypertension or heart diseases step with the left foot first, whereas people with liver diseases step with the right foot first. Cancer patients step the foot of the affected side. Taking stepping the left foot for example, let the heel land the ground first, then by the sole. With the body weight shifting to the left, place the left foot firmly on the ground. Then step with the right foot, let the heel land the ground before the sole. The body weight shifts to the right as the right foot is placed on the ground. As you move ahead step by step, alternate the left and the right. (Figure 4–5 to Figure 4–7)

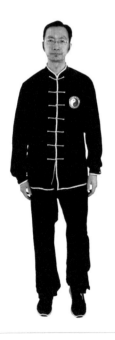

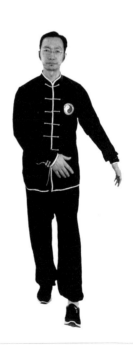

图4-5　Figure 4-5　　　　　图4-6　Figure 4-6

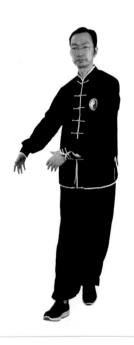

图4-7　Figure 4-7

　　[注意事项]步法要有节奏,要注意松腰、松胯。眼向前方平视(睁眼或闭眼可自行酌定)。要做到"视而不见""听而不闻",以排除外界干扰。同时,舌抵上腭,以沟通任、督二脉。若口津增多,不要边走边咽,等到收功时再咽,以免被呛。头部随身体的扭转而转动,当左脚迈出放平时,身体的重心移至左脚,躯干略向右转,头也随之向右转。转头时要注意放松天柱穴处和后颈、肩等部位。行走的速度及呼吸的长短根据自己的身体状况而定,以轻快不感到憋气为宜。

　　[Notes] Relax the waist and hips and walk in steady paces. Look straight ahead (with eyes closed or open), listen carefully to one's own breathing or rhythmic sounds to remove distractions. Meanwhile, touch the palate with the tongue to connect the Ren and Du meridians. If saliva increases, swallow it after the conclusion to avoid choking. Turn the head with the body. When the left foot touches the ground, the body weight shifts to the left foot and the body and head slightly turn to the right. Relax the area of Tianzhu (BL10), back of the neck and shoulders. The speed and the breathing can be adjusted according to individualized body constitution.

手臂摆动：迈步时手臂的摆动要自然，与迈步配合好。当迈左腿，左足跟轻轻着地时，右手随之摆至中丹田前，左手臂自然向左后侧摆至左胯边。当左脚放平时，随之右脚向前迈进，左手臂由左后侧顺势摆至中丹田前，右手臂自然摆到右胯边。如此左右两脚轮流前行，左右两手也随之自然地前后摆动。（图4-8、图4-9）

Arm swing: Swing the arms naturally while walking. When the left leg is stepped, the left heel gently lands the ground, the right hand swings to the front of the middle Dantian, and the left arm goes to the side of the left hip. When the left foot is level, followed by the right foot forward, swing the left arm to the front of the middle Dantian, the right arm to the side of the right hip. In this way, the feet take turns moving forward, and

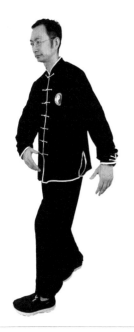
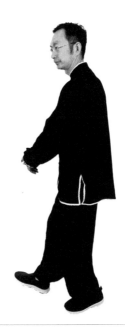

图4-8　Figure 4-8　　　　图4-9　Figure 4-9

the hands also naturally swing back and forth. (Figure 4–8 and Figure 4–9)

［注意事项］当左脚跟着地时，左手臂再开始向左后方摆动，右手向中丹田处摆动，当左脚放平时，右手正对中丹田。手与丹田的位置相距一拳左右。左手正放在左胯边。手摆动与迈步要自然而有节律，不用力，不拿憋劲，肩、肘、腕、全身诸关节均要放松，腋要空虚，臂要保持弧形运动，不要绷直，轻松愉快，所以此功叫作自然行功。

[Notes] When the left foot lands the ground, swing the left arm to the left back and swing the right hand towards the middle Dantian. When the left foot is levelled on the ground, the right hand is facing the middle Dantian. The hands are positioned about a fist away from the Dantian. The left hand is placed at the left hip. The hand swing and step should be natural and rhythmic without using force or holding breath. The shoulders, elbows, wrist and all joints of the body should be relaxed, the armpits should be empty, and the arms should keep an arc movement. This is why this practice is called natural exercise.

2. 调息
2. Breathing Regulation

自然行功的调息方法是风呼吸法。风呼吸法是以鼻呼吸，先吸后呼。吸气时略带"风"声（即气息声），声音大小以自己刚能听到为度，不可太大。吸比呼声短促而略重，呼气声缓而略轻。自然行功的风呼吸法是两吸一呼为一息，即吸、吸、呼。而且呼吸要与步子互相配合。当迈出的左脚，左足跟着地时，马上做两个吸、吸的动作，然后迈出右脚，右足跟着地时再做一个呼的动作。如此吸、吸、呼，吸、吸、呼，一步一步向前行进。

Wind breathing is the technique of breathing through the nose: Inhale first, and then exhale. There is a faint "wind" sound during breathing (i.e. breath sound). The exhalation is long and slight while the inhalation is quick and heavy. In wind breathing, "one breath" is defined as two inhalations accompanied by a single exhalation, that is, inhale, inhale and exhale. The breathing and the movements should be coordinated. One should perform two inhalations as soon as the left foot and heel touch the ground, and then take the right foot and perform an exhalation once the right heel touches the ground. March forward by repeating the sequence of "inhale, inhale and exhale".

［注意事项］两个短"吸"的时间与一个长"呼"的时间基本相等，不可偏长偏短，呼吸节律要自然，气顺神安。如果患有高血压、心脏病者将风呼吸法改为自然呼吸法。

[Notes] The breathing rhythm should be natural with relaxed qi and a calm mind. Two short "inhalations" are equal to one long "exhalation." Patients with heart disease or high blood pressure should change wind breathing to natural breathing.

3. 收功

3. Conclude

行走15分钟后，恢复开始松静站立姿势，站立一会儿后，再做中丹田三开合和3个气呼吸，然后自然松静站立2分钟后慢慢睁开双眼。本功法从预备功开始，行走15分钟，再做简式收功为1段，休息5～10分钟后可以再做1～2段。

After 15 minutes of walking, return to the preparation posture, stand for a while, perform the openings and closings of middle Dantian and 3 times of qi breathing, stand for 2 minutes in a relaxed state and then slowly open the eyes. The exercise begins with preparation posture, followed by a 15-minute walk, and ends by the concluding movement. Repeat after a break of 5–10 minutes.

应用
Application

中度风呼吸法自然行功是运用调息导引法来调整阴阳,调动内气运行,疏通经络脉道,达到防治疾病的目的。具有消炎、祛热、防癌、防病的功效。临床应用范围非常广泛,除严重心脏病外,许多慢性疾病均可采用该法预防和辅助治疗。如肝炎、肺炎、肾炎、肠炎、支气管炎、关节炎、神经衰弱症、感冒发热、月经不调、肺结核、青光眼及其他眼病等均可应用。

Natural qigong exercise in walking with moderate-speed wind-breathing regulates yin and yang, activates internal qi and unblocks meridians by breathing Daoyin. It has anti-inflammatory, antipyretic, anti-cancer and disease-prevention efficacy. Except for severe heart disease, many chronic diseases can be prevented and treated with this exercise, including hepatitis, pneumonia, nephritis, enteritis, bronchitis, arthritis, neurasthenia, fever due to common cold, irregular menstruation, tuberculosis, glaucoma and other eye diseases.

一、二、三步行功是预防和治疗癌症的主要功法。此外对预防感冒和退热、消炎等也有很好的效果。所以该功法很适合于冬季操练，有"过冬功"之称。对肾炎、肝炎、肺炎、气管炎以及肺气肿患者，也可将此功列为主功之一。但严重心绞痛患者不宜操练此功；有轻微心脏病患者操练此功时，呼吸要轻缓柔和或用自然呼吸，动作也要柔和。

Qigong exercise in walking (one, two, or three steps) is considered the main exercise to prevent and deal with cancer. In addition, it also works for common cold, fever and inflammation. As a result, this qigong is often called "winter-friendly qigong". Except for those with severe angina, it is also the main exercise for patients with nephritis, hepatitis, pneumonia, bronchitis, and emphysema. Patients with mild heart disease should breathe slowly, softly or naturally and perform soft movements.

练此功穿衣以轻柔宽大为佳，季节气候变化时，要随时增减衣服，预防感冒。练功时要松开腰带、领口、袖口、表带、穿平底鞋，不穿硬底鞋和高跟鞋。不食辛辣有刺激性食物。清晨练功前，不食或少食一点东西，练完功30分钟后再按常量进食。午后或晚间练功前饭不要吃得太饱，饭后1小时后再练功，功后最少休息30分钟后再做其他事情。安排好练功时间，癌症患者保证每天练功时间不得少于2个小时。

Remember to put on or take off clothes according to weather changes. When performing qigong exercise in walking, one should wear flat shoes, remove the belt, collar, cuffs, and strap, and avoid shoes with firm soles and high heels. Avoid spicy and pungent food. Eat a little or with an empty stomach before morning practice, and then eat after 30 minutes of practice. Avoid overeating before the afternoon or evening practice. It's advisable to exercise 1 hour after eating and to do other jobs 30 minutes after exercise. The practice time should be arranged properly. Cancer patients shall practice for at least 2 hours a day.

五、 内家八卦转掌
Ba Gua (Eight-Diagram) Palm Turning

　　中国功夫无论内家外家都特别注重腿上的功夫，而内家功夫如太极、形意、八卦实际上皆可称为行步功，这里以八卦为代表做简要介绍。八卦掌是内外双修的拳术，它结合了道家的导引吐纳术，融技击、养生、健身于一体，讲内外相合、上下相随、以意领气、以气领力。这种拳术将攻防招数和导引方法融合于绕圆走转之中。讲求纵横交错，随走随练，以变应变，合于《周易》中"刚柔相摩、八卦相荡"、运动不息、变化不止的道理，故名。八卦掌传承于清朝后期的武术宗师董海川，现已传遍全国以及流传遍及全世界。这里主要介绍八卦行步功和八卦转掌走圈功这两种功法。

　　Chinese martial arts, both internal and external, pay extraordinary attention to the exercise of legs and footwork. Internal martial arts, such as Taijiquan, Xing Yi Quan (Form-Intent Fist) and Ba Gua Zhang (Eight-Diagram Palm), all fall under the category of qigong exercise in walking. Here we take Ba Gua Zhang as an example. Ba Gua Zhang emphasizes the cultivation of internal qi as well as physical exercise, featuring palm changes and footwork. Ba Gua Zhang combines Daoyin and breathing of Taoism with combating, health cultivation and bodybuilding. The essence includes combination of internal and external exercise, using intent to guide qi and using qi to guide strength. This technique hides attack and defense within the circular walking movements. The exercise is in line with the theory of "combination of softness and strength and overlapping of the eight diagrams" in the *Yi Jing* (Book of Changes), it was therefore named as "Ba Gua Zhang". Ba Gua Zhang was devised by Master Dong Haichuan in the late Qing Dynasty, and has spread all over China and the world. Here we will introduce Ba Gua (Eight-Diagram) Walking and Ba Gua Palm Turning and Circular Walking.

（一）八卦行步功
Ba Gua (Eight-Diagram) Qigong Exercise in Walking

　　转掌功是八卦掌重要的核心基本功法之一，代表了八卦掌的拳术特点。若要练好八卦转掌，就应先练好行步功。行步功的习练是为了锻炼好初习者的腰腿力量及行步时的平衡能力和稳定性，为下一步练转掌打下坚实的基础，给八大掌、六十四掌、游身八卦连环掌的学习做铺垫。

Palm turning encapsulates and symbolizes Ba Gua Zhang's characteristics. Qigong exercise in walking can strengthen the lower body, improve the walking stability and balance, and serve as the foundation for Ba Da Zhang, Liu Shi Si Zhang (Sixty-four Palm) and Ba Gua Palm Turning and You Shen Ba Gua Lian Huan Zhang (Swimming Dragon Eight Diagram Palm).

　　行步功与转掌不同，它属于直行的练功方法，看似简单易学，但真要按照要求去做的话，初时还是很吃功夫的。在八卦转掌功夫里走的蹚泥步，绕圈圆转时做摆扣步法，初习者由于缺乏腰腿功夫，会出现左摇右摆等现象，因而要达到蹚泥步中平起平落的走步，一般是不容易的。但若习练行步功后，如能持之以恒、循序渐进的话，练出了腰腿及步法上的功夫后，再进一步练习转掌的蹚泥步时，就相对容易些，从而起到事半功倍的作用。

Unlike palm turning, qigong exercise in walking seems easy; however, it takes a lot of time and efforts. Due to insufficient strength in the waist and legs, beginners may experience swaying of the upper body while practicing mud-wading walking. Persistent exercise will gradually make things easier.

据称，此功是由山东陈济生先生所传，当年上海的殷继成先生曾撰文做过介绍。

According to a paper written by Mr. Yin Jicheng from Shanghai, this practice was handed down by Mr. Chen Jisheng (1904–1988) from Shandong Province.

操作要领
Tips

1. 调身
1. Body Regulation

起势：两脚并拢，立正开始，全身放松，自然站立，双掌松垂体侧，掌指向下，两肩两臂放松，头正颈直，微收下颏，舌抵上腭，呼吸自然，用鼻呼吸，上身正直，双目平视前方。略微调息片刻，待心平气和之后，双臂外旋，变掌心向下，经面向前慢慢下落至腹前，双掌在腹前下按，两手指相对，中指相平呈一线，两大拇指微靠于丹田处，两臂开成环形，同时呼气松腹，气沉于丹田，腹部微外突，肛微上提，两脚不动，随双掌下垂微屈膝下蹲，此势可站立几分钟。(图5-1、图5-2)

Starting posture: Place the feet together, keep the body upright, relax the body, stand naturally, drop the hands to the

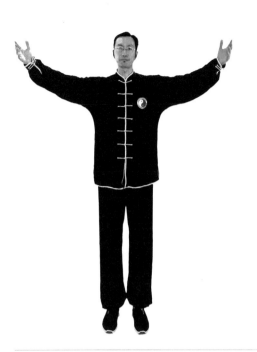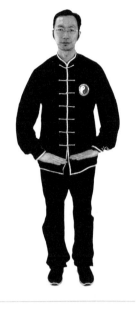

图5-1　Figure 5-1　　　　　图5-2　Figure 5-2

sides with fingertips pointing downward, relax the shoulders and arms, slightly tuck the chin in, touch the palate with the tongue, breathe naturally with the nose, and look straight ahead. Regulate the breathing, tranquilize the mind, and turn the arms outward. Then with the palms pointing downward, press the palms down in front of the abdomen with the fingers of both hands facing each other, and put two thumbs slightly against the Dantian. Open the arms in a circle, relax the abdomen, and exhale. Sink qi down to the Dantian, slightly lift up the anus, don't move the feet, and slightly bend the knees as the palms drop down. Keep the posture for a few minutes. (Figure 5–1 and Figure 5–2)

［注意事项］两臂开成环形时，两肘尖外撑圆，但不可用力，要放松。臀向后坐、内敛，头正身直，有虚领顶劲之势，双目向前平视，此势可站立几分钟。待精力充沛，丹田处有气息充实，有

鼓荡之感时，再行下一势。

[Notes] When opening the arms in a circle, extend the elbows naturally outward (do not use force). Put the body weight on the buttocks, keep the body and head upright as if a string is holding you up from above, look straight ahead, and stand in this posture for a few minutes. Start the next movement when you feel energetic and the Dantian is full of qi.

将重心移至右脚上，左脚不抬，足跟轻轻提起，微离地面，但不可过高，收至右脚踝内侧，此时左脚脚底仍有与地面微蹭的相接之感。然后左腿放松向前缓缓迈步蹚出。（图5-3、图5-4）

Place the body weight on the right foot, slightly lift the left heel above the ground, and move the left foot to the medial aspect of the right ankle. Then, relax the left leg and slowly take a step forward. (Figure 5-3 and Figure 5-4)

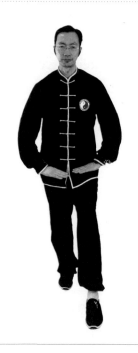 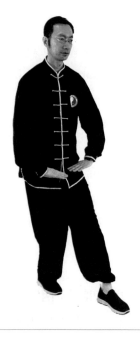

图5-3　Figure 5-3　　　　　图5-4　Figure 5-4

［注意事项］脚尖不可上翘抬起，至脚面伸直时，脚面绷直，劲力达于脚趾，趾尖微扣，但身高不变，不可迈步前进而有起伏，后脚仍呈微下蹲之势，两掌仍在腹前呈平按掌，头正身直，勿左右歪斜。初习之时会出现身动腿抖的现象，待练日久功深之后，自然会腿部有力，站立平稳。

[Notes] Do not lift up the toes, slightly turn the toes downward and move steadily while the height of the body remains the same. When moving, keep the back leg slightly bent, press the palms in front of the abdomen and at the same time, keep the body and head upright. Beginners may experience shaking legs and body moving due to insufficient leg strength. With persistent practice, one may stand steadily.

做脚下步法上的虚实转换，将左脚落地踏实，五趾微抓地。胯与膝均放松向前缓缓移动重心向左腿上，左腿由虚变实，后腿渐虚伸直，呈左弓步之势。

Shift the weighted and unweighted footstep. When the left foot lands on the ground, slightly grasp the ground with the toes, relax the hips and knees, and then slowly shift the body weight from the right leg to the left leg to form a left bow step.

［注意事项］向前进时身体不可高起或下蹲，保持高度如前。

[Notes] Keep your body upright as you move forward. Avoid stooping or tiptoeing.

仍保持头正身直，身体高度如前，气向下沉，微提肛，全身放松，用腰胯之力平提后脚向前上步，提步全凭腰胯及重心向右脚下踩之力运动。右脚收至左脚踝内侧，两足平行相并，但右脚不可着地，只左脚单脚着地站立，呈独立式，双掌仍平按于丹田处，臀部内敛，肛微上提，双目仍前视。(图5-5、图5-6)

Keep the head and body upright, sink qi down to the Dantian, slightly lift the anus, relax the whole body, and lift the right foot for a step forward using the strength of the waist and hips. Lift the right foot up to the medial aspect of the left ankle. Put the feet together, with only the left foot standing on the ground. Press the palms in front of the Dantian. Tuck in the buttocks, slightly lift the anus and look straight ahead. (Figure 5-5 and Figure 5-6)

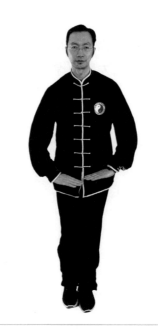

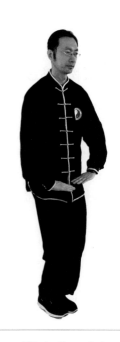

图5-5　Figure 5-5　　　　　图5-6　Figure 5-6

[注意事项] 提脚不可高，如在地面上拖着一般前蹚，脚跟不可抬起，脚底仍与地面相平，提步时身勿前俯用力，也不可抬高身体来带动后脚前提，下颏微收，头不可后仰。

[Notes] Slightly lift the foot with the heel touching the

ground. Avoid pulling your torso up to lift your foot or bringing your foot forward by leaning forwards. Keep the head up and slightly tuck the chin in.

右脚如左脚般向前蹬出，向前平伸迈步蹬出，脚面伸直，劲力达于脚趾上，高度为微离地面，再向前踏实，将腰胯前移成右弓步，再用腰胯劲提左脚向前并步，右脚独立站立，其要领行功均与左势相同。如此反复，向前迈出蹬出，行走练习。(图5-7～图5-10)

Step the right foot forward like the left, with the right heel touching the ground and the right toes slightly grasping the ground. Then shift the weighted step onto the right foot, and slowly shift the body weight from the left leg to the right leg to form a right bow step. Lift the left foot for a step forward using the strength of the waist and hips. Put the feet together, with only the right foot standing on the ground. The requirements

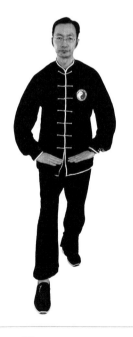

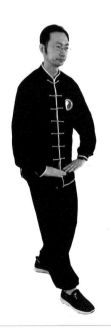

图5-7   Figure 5-7   图5-8   Figure 5-8

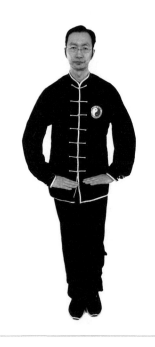 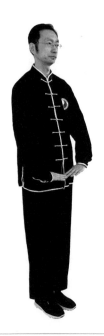

图5-9　Figure 5-9　　　　　　　　图5-10　Figure 5-10

are the same as before. Repeat the procedures and practice stepping the foot forward. (Figure 5–7 to Figure 5–10)

［注意事项］行步时脚要平起平落, 有如履薄冰之感, 练习不拘步数及时间。此功亦可在练习时将双掌先收至丹田处, 两掌指相对平按腹部前, 再双臂外旋, 变成两掌自然收至两胯旁, 掌心向下或掌指自然向下松垂体侧, 然后再做迈步向前平蹚的行步之功, 如此则上身及双臂不会那么紧张或用力过多。

[Notes] Slightly lift the foot off the ground with the heel touching the ground when walking, just like walking on an ice lake. The movement can be practiced without limitations on steps or duration. Beginners can use adjusted movements. For example, one can press the palms down in front of the abdomen, extend the arms outward, and then drop the arms to the sides of the body with the fingers pointing downward. In this way, the upper body and arms will not tense up or overuse force.

应注意初练之时, 会出现身体因腰腿的劲力而致平衡能力不够, 产生左摇右摆和腿上颤抖, 或前俯后仰, 腰腿酸痛, 呼吸不匀等现象。因此需用心练习, 行步时五趾可用力微抓地, 以增强其稳定能力, 行走时不可过快, 上身及迈步之腿均要放松, 身体不要上下起伏, 后脚向前进时勿拔跟。待功力深后, 自然会迈步平稳, 腰腿有力。练功中周身会出现发热或出汗, 应及时将汗擦干勿吹风, 还应该注意减少房事。口中有津液要保持咽下, 以意送至丹田处。

Due to the weak waist and leg muscles, beginners may experience body swaying, soreness, uneven breathing, or leg shaking. They can try grasping the ground with toes when walking to maintain balance, keeping the upper body and legs relaxed when walking forward, always keeping the heels on the ground. One will naturally walk steadily as their legs and waist become stronger over time. During exercise, one may experience feverish sensation or sweating. It is necessary to wipe up the sweat, avoid exposure to wind and reduce the frequency of sex. When saliva starts to produce, swallow them and sink them down to the Dantian using the intent.

2. 调息
2. Breathing Regulation

习练本功法时, 保持自然呼吸, 以自然逆腹式呼吸可达到气沉丹田的作用。

Breathe naturally when practicing. Performing reverse abdominal breathing may help sink qi down to the Dantian.

3. 调心

3. Mind Regulation

习练时收心内敛,保持静心状态,行步时意识关注两脚的虚
实变化。

Keep the mind undistracted when practicing. Concentrate on
the weighted and unweighted shifting of both feet while walking.

应用
Application

本功法是八卦转掌的基本功,久习可以祛病健身强身,增加
腿部的力量与平衡性,也可为进一步习练八卦转掌打下一定的
基础。

This movement is a basic exercise for Ba Gua (Eight-
Diagram) Palm Turning. Long-time exercise can strengthen the
body as well as improve leg strength and balance.

(二)八卦转掌
Ba Gua (Eight-Diagram) Palm Turning

八卦掌以"行桩""蹚泥步"内功功法为入门基础,以拧翻
走转为基本运动形式,以掌法的变化为主要技击手段。内外兼
修,强调身心合练,身捷步灵如故龙游空,拧翻走转掌法幻变无
穷。出手成招,刚柔相济,踢打摔拿融为一体。拧裹钻翻,避正
打斜,围圆打点,循循相生无有穷尽。

Ba Gua Zhang integrates internal and external exercise,

combines softness with hardness, and features flexible and diverse motions. It takes "moving stances" and "mud-wading walking" as basic internal exercises and palm turning as well as footwork as basic movements. The circling walking is interconnected as a series of continuous movements by kicking, punching, wrestling, and gripping.

习练蹚泥步由开始蹚不出去步,练到蹚出去而又稳健。蹚泥步利于气往下沉,主要练习重心的水平移动,它比形意的直线水平移动要难,因为它要走圈,人体的重心要在一个水平的圆圈上移动。八卦步练好了,自然会融会贯通,重心要向不同方向的水平移动也就不难了。能够把重心水平地向着一个方向移动,并把整体重量输送到一点上,从而得到很好的打击效果。站架行桩,内守中定,外重八要,身动意不变,如水漂木,一气流行。先练直蹚泥步,练的蹚步平稳了再练走圈蹚泥步,然后学练站八卦桩,而后再学练掌。

Mud-wading walking can help sink qi down to the Dantian, and the key is to change the body weight and move in a horizontal circle on the basis of Ba Gua footwork. This allows the force to be focused on a single point and exerted with the palms, producing a tremendous strike. With the emphasis on post-standing exercises and moving stances, the practitioner should walk with a focused mind, like driftwood on the water, combining motion and stillness. Beginners should first practice straight and circular mud-wading walking, followed by the Ba Gua stance and Ba Gua Zhang.

站桩是八卦掌转掌走圈的基础和精髓,坚持下来会觉得身体特别舒服有劲,两脚如植地生根,站着站着觉得有一种顶天立地的气势和万夫不挡的勇气,越站越爱站。等待对方发球前的那一刻的身体状态,蓄而待发,肌肉的松紧状态,不软也不僵,富含撑裹劲又弹性十足,这种状态就是站八卦桩所要具备的东西,这样练一段时间启动速度会非常快。

Ba Gua Zhang's circular mud-wading walking exercise is built on post-standing exercise. After a long period of practice, the body becomes strong with sufficient internal qi, the muscles are relaxed and full of elastic force, and the state during exercise is like a goalkeeper waiting for the ball, preparing to move at any time.

转圈将基本功和最高层功夫统一成极简单、内涵又极丰富的练功方法,是八卦特有的劲力与身法相结合的方法。是在不断的盘旋绕转中,仍然能够身体放松,脑子精神安静舒适,然后再静中求动达到专一而不乱。能产生一种旋涡让习者能将其放大、混合、控制,自然能量透过自身与天地往来,这种拧转的作用根据练者心意产生螺旋能波,同时这种能也可反过来带动其形气,在高级阶段,此旋涡可同时飞腾于天及沉降于地,并产生威力惊人的杀伤破坏效果。球状或弧状能承受更强的压力,也可通过螺旋积极的转换或偏转能量,要精通这种技巧,应用意而不是用力来完成。

Circular walking, a unique technique for combining strength and body movements in Ba Gua Zhang, integrates basic movements with advanced exercise as a simple but ever-changing exercise. The practice can help the body and mind become peaceful and relaxed and reach a focused state. As a result, the spiral energy wave is generated, and the natural energy from heaven and earth can communicate with the body through the practitioner's mind, and this energy can in turn drive the form of qi. In the advanced stage, the spiral energy wave can soar into the sky or settle down to the ground, causing massive destruction. To be proficient in this technique, it should be done with intention rather than force.

转圈把"意、气、力"三方面有机地糅合在一起,在连贯圆活的肢体运动中达到外动内静,意气相随的境地,气沉而不浮,归于丹田,久久加功,精神与肢体都可获得最高的呼应。临敌格斗,一触即发,其产生的强大内劲猛不可挡,有如电力,顷刻之间,可置敌于寻丈之外。久久习练渐渐达到行步如蹚泥,全身不滞不散,不迟不断,腰似车轴,气如行云。换式如高山流水,连绵不断。两脚要虚实分明,左右互移。抽身换形,翻若惊鸿,随机应变,奥妙无穷。

Through circular walking, "intent," "qi," and "strength" are interconnected via roundness and continuous body movements. During the exercise, the intent flows with qi, and the qi sinks down to the Dantian. With long-term exercise, the mind and body can all be strengthened, stepping forward is like walking in muddy places, with the internal qi circulating through continuous movements and footwork. As a result, the internal strength is unstoppable, as fast as electricity, and can defeat the enemy a dozen steps away.

操作要领
Tips

行步是蹚泥步的基础,练习行步之后再走圈,会有事半功倍的效果。

Walking practice is the basis of circular mud-wading walking.

1. 调身
1. Body Regulation

走圈——圆形蹚泥步
Circular walking

（1）身体保持中正，放松，沉肩坠肘、含胸拔背等。

(1) Keep the body relaxed and upright, sink the shoulders and drop the elbows, tuck in the chest and pull up the back.

（2）双掌下按至丹田处，意如按水中浮木。

(2) Like pressing a piece of floating wood in the water, press the hands down to the Dantian.

（3）屈膝下蹲至适宜高度。

(3) Bend the knees and slightly squat down.

（4）左手转掌心向上，从右前臂下穿出，经右前方穿向身体左侧，掌心向外，高与肩齐，右掌按于腹部左侧，掌心斜向下，身体和腰部略向左拧转。同时左脚略向右前方蹚出，接着重心移向左腿，右脚贴地向前蹚出，脚尖内扣向左。

(4) Move the left hand through the right forearm with the palm facing up, then move it to the left side of the body to the shoulder level with the palm facing out. With hands down, gently press the right palm in front of the left abdomen. Turn your body and waist a bit to the left. Step out with the left foot

slightly to the right front at the same moment. After that, put the body weight on the left leg. Step out with the right foot, with the toes pointing left.

（5）左右胯重心相互转换，绕圈逆时针蹚步而行。

(5) As you walk counterclockwise around the circle, alternately place your body weight on the left and right hips.

（6）摩膝蹚胫，脚掌平起平落。（图5-11～图5-17）

(6) Practice the mud-wading walk with small steps that entail knees rubbing against each other and feet touching the ground. (Figure 5-11 to Figure 5-17)

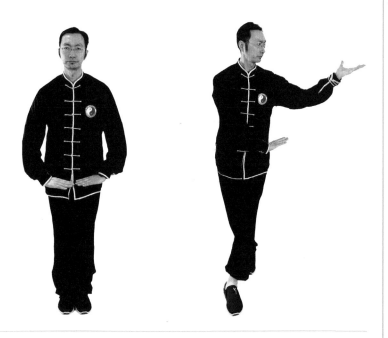

图5-11　Figure 5-11　　　　图5-12　Figure 5-12

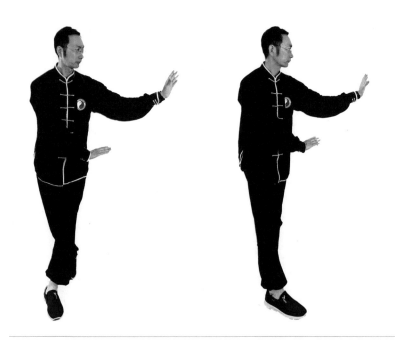

图5-13　Figure 5-13　　　　图5-14　Figure 5-14

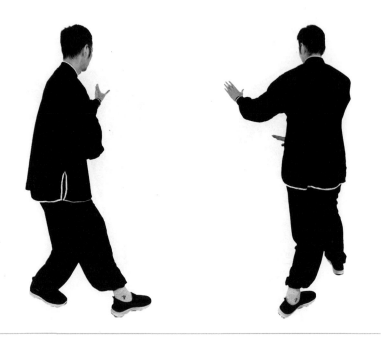

图5-15　Figure 5-15　　　　图5-16　Figure 5-16

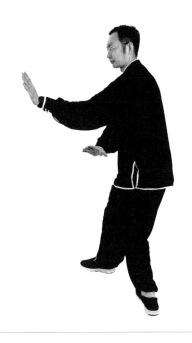

图5-17　Figure 5-17

（7）以上为左式，右式动作同上，唯方向相反。中间须通过移行换步连接。（图5-18～图5-23）

(7) The above is the counterclockwise circling, and the clockwise circling is the same as the above, but in the opposite

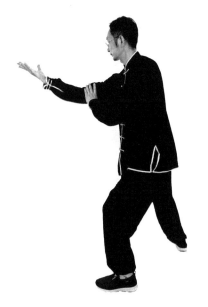

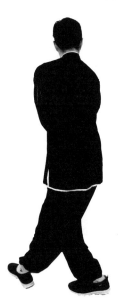

图5-18　Figure 5-18　　　　　图5-19　Figure 5-19

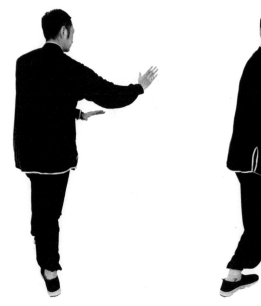
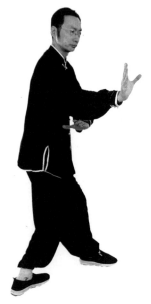

图5-20　Figure 5-20　　　　图5-21　Figure 5-21

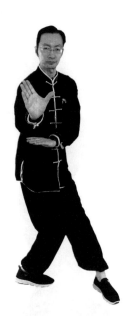
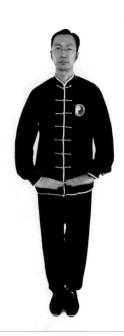

图5-22　Figure 5-22　　　　图5-23　Figure 5-23

direction. The movements are connected through moving and changing steps. (Figure 5–18 to Figure 5–23)

2. 调息
2. Breathing Regulation

呼吸任其自然，气自然往下沉。

Breathe naturally and allow qi to sink down.

3. 调心
3. Mind Regulation

初学时，意念稍注于足底涌泉穴，此为要诀。意念上有松沉的意境，日久气沉涌泉，乃至地心。

It's advisable for beginners to concentrate their minds on Yongquan (KI1). With the mind's concentration, qi in the body can relax and descend to the feet.

注意事项
Notes

走圈最好能转树，通过以树为圆心的不断走转，才练就出腰如轴立的横劲。转树功法的根本目的是练腿和腰，腰如轴立不是孤立的，其基础还在腿，而且是运动着的腿，走起来要稳如坐轿，才能发挥腰部拧转的劲力，才能将这股螺旋劲上达臂掌，所以走是根本的根本。

It is preferable to circle a tree: By moving continuously and using the tree as the pivot, one can strengthen the transverse strength of the waist. This exercise aims to strengthen the waist and legs together, since the strength of the waist relies on the strength of the legs, especially moving legs. In order to transfer the waist strength to the arms and palms, walking should be as stable as sitting on a palanquin. Walking is, therefore, the most basic of all.

练走圈并不是一上来就要转树,先学会步法并标准化,然后走直蹚并垂臂,等腿上有劲稳定了自然了再走圈,这时先走大圈,脚微微内扣,慢慢地再收缩,等腿完全变稳,如坐轿了,然后才拧腰转树走八式。初练时先走大圈,上身拧转不要过大,否则腰不活,硬往里拧,走转不稳,心火上升,内气不调,五脏会受损。

Learning correct footwork is the first step in practicing circular walking. Then practice straight walking with the arms dropped until the legs are strong enough. After that, you can start walking in a circle. Walk in a big circle first, slightly bending the toes inward. Over time, you can walk in a smaller circle. After the legs are strong enough (like sitting on a palanquin) and you can walk steadily, you can practice tree-circling accompanied by the waist rotating. Same as before, walk in a big circle first with slight rotation to avoid internal qi disharmony, ascending of heart fire and impairment of the five-zang organs.

初练时走转要慢,由慢到快,可早练慢,晚练快,不可操之过急。要想功力增长快,慢练是最好的途径,在功力训练一定时间以后,还要同时练习身法,快练主要以步法配合身法,以身法找步法,以步法身法带动掌法变化。

At first, beginners should move slowly. Or they can practice slow walking in the morning and fast walking in the evening.

Persistent practice is the best way to make progress. Over time, the practice should emphasize posture and body movements too. During the fast-walking practice, the footwork is connected with body movements. The two are as crucial as the footwork because they are linked to the palms turning.

转圈有快慢之分,快转锻炼身法、步法、眼法,久转之使身法非常灵活,练的是腿脚身法。慢练也叫细练,功效是出内功,练的是内气,着重练气,逐步体会阴阳虚实的转换(胯),应该越慢越不嫌慢,配合呼吸,应比打太极还慢,始终是用一只脚在支撑体重,找横劲,要用丹田领着走。

Circular walking can be fast or slow. Fast circular walking exercises body movements, footwork and eyes. Slow circular walking focuses on internal exercise and can strengthen internal qi. The slow circular walking involves the transition of yin, yang and body weight. Assisted by breathing, the walking pace is slower than Taiji. The body weight always falls on one leg, and the Dantian strength propels the body forward while walking.

刚练时是慢的,可以说是一种暗劲儿,是慢慢地小心地蹚,慢慢找出这股劲。从走中求身劲的整,求出了内家的整和顺。随着功夫日益渐长,步子越长身架就越低。走圈能使全身上下协调一致。

The walking exercise develops overall strength and moves at a slow pace at the beginning. Over time, the stride may grow longer, and the posture may get lower. Walking in circles can synchronize the body as a whole.

八卦掌左旋右转,以斜打正,处处走圆,走圈功就能练出圆

脚平起平落随着掌法的变化。行功是要在如痴如醉的轻缓步态
中体会天人合一、无人无我的境界。

Ba Gua Zhang features body turning, circular walking and angled palming. Circular walking exercises can develop circular footwork. During the exercise, the body moves steadily with each step and palm change. By walking slowly, softly, and with a flexible posture, walking exercise of Ba Gua Zhang can achieve a state of man-nature unity.

走圈过程中不能休息中断，如换式也应如太极般一手接一手其势连绵不断，一气练下去，不可中断，断则散。每次练习的时候如果能走到一百圈的运动量或者确保半小时，这样就比较容易有气沉丹田的充实感，而且全身的劲、气流动也会让人感到运动后的舒畅，双手会感到充满劲力。

Circular walking should be practiced all at once, with no breaks or interruptions, because interruptions will scatter qi. The posture change is continuous, like Taiji Tui Shou (Taiji Palm). It is recommended to walk for 100 laps or 30 minutes at a time. Because in this way it is easier to feel a sensation of qi fullness in the Dantian, and qi is circulating throughout the entire body. As a result, you will feel comfortable, and subsequently, your hands are full of strength.

转圈是架势使然，如果架势没有拧转的动力而勉强走圈，是未得要领。当深入八卦高层后，会发觉不得不转，在于全身各部位的拧转，当八卦拳的架势出来之后，会带动出一个行动力，形成了前进的势和拧转的势，实际上是劲在走。最初是身体产生势，后来是整个势在带动身体，单换掌要掌握那个势，身体要随势而走。转掌到后来不是走的，而是被身形逼出来的，所有的招

式都兼带反弹力，身法步法全都是在别劲中进行，要将腰的柔韧性练习到像一条龙一样，几乎盘在树上。

By following the movements, you will naturally walk in a circle. Especially when you enter the advanced stage of Ba Gua exercises, the circling and rotating drive all body parts. The movements of Ba Gua Zhang will cause the body to advance and walk in a circle. It is the internal strength that causes the walking. The body develops its internal strength first and then moves in accordance with it. The waist is flexible while walking in a circle, like a dragon coiling around a tree.

八卦的进退是借身形架构的轻微改变而改变架势的势，所以是身随势，步随身。不是用腿去迈，而是用整个身形催动腿走出。等到丹田气足，催动全身，则走转会越来越快。初练时走的圈要大一些，会走大圈的人也会走小圈。有功夫后，可以走大圈也可以走小圈。大圈练习力气，小圈练习功夫，初练圈要不大不小，方便找劲，入门后圈要小方便长劲。

Rather than a simple forward or backward step, the forward and backward movements of the body are driven by a change in posture. Sufficient qi in the Dantian will propel the body to walk faster in a circle. When beginners have mastered the movements, they can opt to walk in a small circle. Initially, they can walk in a large circle. While walking in a small circle develops internal qi and strength, walking in a large circle enhances qi and strength.

转掌眼神闪烁不定会让意念跑掉，意念要守在内。脊骨要会上下呼吸，不是用外力去使力使劲，而是用意用脊骨内息驱动着整个人体，一个起心动念内息马上在脊骨运作一上一下地做内呼吸，转掌练的就是脊骨中的内息运作的任督两脉做小周天循环，进而练就深厚的内功。其快是因为意念比敌人快，内息通畅无碍。走转时讲究左右平衡，特别是内功掌，左右转的圈数应该基本相当，否则导致左右半身气血循环失调，左右半身会一边冷一边热。

It is essential to control the mental concentration during palm turning. The spine should breathe up and down naturally (via the *Ren* and *Du* meridians) instead of being pulled up or down by external force. Intention controls the spine's internal breathing. The Ba Gua (Eight-Diagram) Palm Turning aims to create a small heavenly circle by unblocking the *Ren* and *Du* meridians in the spine. Because the palm is driven by intention, it strikes quickly. Intention is undoubtedly faster than physical movement. Circular walking emphasizes the balance of the left and right, that is, walking the same number of laps in both directions; otherwise, it will cause disharmony of qi and blood circulating in the left and right body parts, leading to a hot sensation on one side and a cold sensation on the other side.

行到极佳处，即忘其行；达到行功如站功，动功如静功，实是在动中求静而至真静，故仍归回静功。走转起来即要有随天而运、随地而行之悠悠，又要有神充天地、意满环宇之气势。时时势势要呼吸绵绵，自自然然。走到日月星辰亦与我同旋转；又如站三体式桩，直站到山川河岳与我同呼吸；再如太极拳，一举动则我之开合天地亦与我同开合，是天人合一，是人与自然的协调。

By entering an advanced state, one may forget that he is walking. Walking movements, standing movements, motion, and stillness are all merged and interlinked. That is, to walk with the rhythm of nature, symbolize the vigor of the universe, and rotate with the moon and stars. The breathing is natural, soft and continuous, like in San Ti Shi (Heaven-Earth-Human) standing exercises. The movements are coherent, like Taijiquan, featuring the harmony between man and nature.

转圈发展平衡力和敏感度,也是发展速度和力量的基础。练套路虽可增加功力,但绝不能代替转圈,八卦的特点通过转圈的习练都可达到。八卦的各个掌式,都有其左旋右转的劲力变换方式,通了这个劲力变换,转圈几乎就是八卦的一切,练功与散手都含在其中。

Circular walking helps to develop the balance ability and sensitivity, which are the basis for speed and strength. The practice of martial arts routines may boost strength, but it cannot take the role of circular walking. Circular walking can help one acquire Ba Gua's features. Palm turning styles in Ba Gua Zhang have their own unique patterns of strength change via circular walking, including routine movements and San Shou (Free Hand).

应用
Application

八卦掌是传统内家功夫之一,习练后可以修养身心,祛病健身,日久功深还能成就内家功夫。通过不断的习练能够开筋通络,增强内气以修成内功,同时锻炼筋骨皮肉,最后达到内外兼修、强身健体的功用。

Ba Gua Zhang is a form of traditional internal martial arts. It can cultivate the body and mind, eliminate disease, and strengthen the body. Through persistent practice, it can unblock meridians, enhance the internal energy to cultivate internal strength, and at the same time, strengthen the bones and muscles, finally exercising both the interior and exterior and benefiting the health.

附：步罡踏斗
Appendix: Bu Gang Ta Dou (Big Dipper Walking)

步罡踏斗是道家著名的以行步为主要行式的修炼功法，据传能沟通天地的能量与信息用以修炼自身。但此功法一般均在道家各派内部流传，外界少有流传。现摘录部分以供大家观摩与参考，但如未得正式传授，请不要轻易尝试练习。

As an exercise for Taoists, Bu Gang Ta Dou (Big Dipper Walking) is a form of walking cultivation. It is said that it can communicate the energy of heaven and earth to cultivate oneself. However, this technique is only circulated within the Taoist schools. Here are some of the excerpts for reference. Do not try to practice them unless you have a good tutor.

天罡七星步
Tian Gang Qi Xing Bu (Seven Stars Walking)

在踏七星步前，要先熟练掌握以下基本步法、基本手法和呼吸方法以及熟记口诀，然后再开始正式练习。

Before the practice of Tian Gang Qi Xing Bu (Seven Stars Walking), first master the following basic footwork, movements and breathing pattern as well as memorize the formula.

1. 预备式

1. Preparation Movement

习练者自然松静站立,两手自然下垂,闭目合齿,舌抵上腭。调整到自然呼吸,呼吸要求匀、深、细、长,使呼吸形成规律。随后再归炁于下丹田,踏步入七星。七星阵如图5-24所示。

Stand in relaxation and tranquility with separated feet, drop the arms naturally to the sides, close the eyes and mouth, and touch the palate with the tongue. Adjust to natural

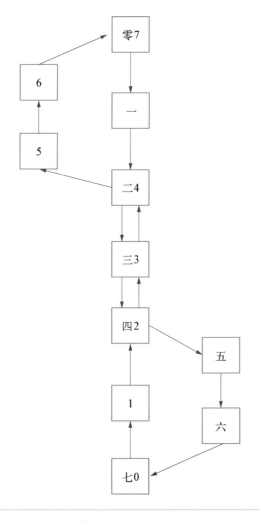

图5-24　Figure 5-24

breathing. The breathing should be even, soft and deep. Then, sink qi down to the lower Dantian and walk along the seven stars in sequence (the seven positions as shown in Figure 5–24).

2. 步法
2. Footwork

从0位开始,左脚拖地向前蹚,左脚落1位后,右脚再拖地向前蹚到,到2位,如此向前走,左脚到3、5位,右脚到4、6位,左脚踏到7位后,右脚也并到7位(两脚稍分开一点,即右脚到7位旁的0位),此时,转体180°,左脚反过来再踏一、三、五位,右脚踏二、四、六位,左脚到七位,右脚也到七位,再转体180°,继续做,如此循环反复。

Standing on "0," step the left foot to "1" with the heel touching the ground, then the right foot to "2" with the heel touching the ground. Continue with the left foot at "3" and "5" and the right foot at "4" and "6". When the left foot lands on "7", step the right foot to "7", and then put the feet together. After that, turn around and continue walking on the same numbers as before, and repeat the procedures.

3. 手法
3. Body Movements

两手置于胸前,十指尖向上,两掌心相对,两臂向左右两侧展开,同时,两手立掌向外推,推至八成时,两手转掌,掌心相对,开始向中间挤压,到两手快要接触时,两手再转掌,掌心向外推,如此循环。在两手由向里压转成向外分手和由分手转成向里压时,转换动作要干净利落,越快越好。

Put both hands in front of the chest with ten fingers pointing upward and two palms facing each other. Keep the palms upright and push outward, when the arms are pushed 80% outward, turn the palms facing each other, and then push inward. When two palms are about to touch each other, turn the palms, and push outward (as ① – ④ shown in Figure 5–25). Repeat the above procedures. The palm turning should be as fast as possible.

4. 呼吸
4. Breathing

呼气时两手向外分,吸气时两手向内压,两掌开合配呼吸。

The opening and closing of the palms correspond to breathing. Exhale when pushing the palms outward and inhale when pushing the palms inward.

5. 收功
5. Conclude

回到0位后,调整自然呼吸片刻,即可收功。

Go back to "0" and adjust to natural breathing to conclude.

注意事项
Notes

（1）整个步法,要求神与意合,意与气合。

(1) Mind-intent unity and intent-qi unity are required during walking.

（2）练天罡七星步的时间是夜间子时，因为子时肾中生炁，合于七星修炼，效果最好。其他时间最好别练。

(2) It's better to practice Tian Gang Qi Xing Bu (Seven Stars Walking) at 11∶00 p.m. At that time, the kidney will generate internal qi. It is in line with the cultivation of the seven stars. Don't practice at other time.

（3）踏在星位上的脚和脚跟不要抬起来，这就要求两腿必须下蹲，下蹲的幅度量力而行。

(3) Don't lift the foot or heel in the star position (numbers in Figure 5−24), which requires slightly bending the knees.

（4）出步时，脚是拖地往前蹚，踏入星位时，是蹭地入位。

(4) When moving the feet, keep the heels or tiptoes touching the ground.

（5）呼吸是先呼后吸，先用鼻呼鼻吸，再进一步就用鼻吸口呼。

(5) For breathing, exhale first, and then inhale. First, exhale and inhale through your nose. Gradually, inhale through your nose and exhale through your mouth.

（6）两掌外掰时呼气，内压时吸气，反之会出现胸闷，身体不舒服。

(6) Exhale when pushing the palms outward, and inhale when pushing the palms inward. Otherwise, chest tightness or discomfort may occur.

（7）要想使人体作为一个整体与七星相联系，踏步时的动作和形态必须做到家，即要做出它的神韵来。用形象化来比喻：

(7) To associate the human body with seven stars, the movement and body posture must be as vivid as follows:

手如雁：手要像大雁一样飘然悠闲，掌要挺直，腕要灵活。

Hand like a goose: The hand movements should be as leisurely as those of a goose, with extended palms and flexible wrists.

背如熊：得做出熊浑厚、稳重的形象。

Back like a bear: Imitate a bear's thick and steady back.

脚如鸵鸟：脚像鸵鸟一样在地下蹚着走。

Foot like an ostrich: Moving like an ostrich in desert, with heels touching the sand.

足如鹤：足吊起来就像鹤一样。

Foot like a crane: The foot hangs up, just like a crane.

体如白云：体态如白云那样轻盈飘逸。

Body like white clouds: The body posture is as light and soft as white clouds.

行 步 功 ● *Xing Bu Gong* (Qigong Exercise in Walking)

Application

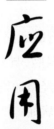

行步功属于传统气功导引功法之一,通过各种行走的训练,配合呼吸、意识的运用,有如下的功效与作用。

Qigong exercise in walking falls under the category of traditional Daoyin exercise. Through various walking exercises combined with breathing and intent regulation, it has the following benefits.

疏通经络
Unblock Meridians

经络是气血运行的通路。经络不通则痛,脏腑组织器官得不到气血的滋养和温煦,导致各种病症。通过行步功的习练可有效促进经络疏通,经络通则不痛,脏腑组织就能得到气血的供应,减轻或消除各种病症。

Meridians are the pathways for qi and blood circulation. Blockage of meridians causes pain and malnourishment of zang-fu organs and tissues. This exercise can unblock meridians, increase qi and blood supply to the zang-fu organs and tissues, and thus alleviate or eliminate disorders or diseases.

调和气血
Harmonize Qi and Blood

气血是滋养人体的营养物质。如果气血不足就可导致贫血或营养不良，免疫功能下降，产生虚症；如果气滞血瘀就可导致气血运行障碍，产生实证。通过习练行步功，能增强腿脚的实力，长劲、长气、长力，不仅可以补益气血，而且又可理气活血，所以能够防治虚症和实证的许多病症。

Qi and blood nurture the body. Insufficient qi and blood may cause anemia, malnutrition, weakened immune system and deficiency syndrome. Qi stagnation and blood stasis may cause excess syndrome. This exercise can strengthen the legs and feet, supplement and regulate qi, promote the circulation of blood. As a result, it can be used for both deficiency syndrome and excess syndrome.

祛病健身

Remove Diseases and Promote Health

通过长期的行步功锻炼既可扶助正气，又可祛除邪气，能够起到祛病健身的作用，长期习练本功法能调理三焦、疏肝、健脾，对虚症内脏下垂、高血压、肠胃病、便秘、内分泌失调以及免疫功能低下等病症有较好的防治作用。可防治虚症内脏下垂、肠胃病、便秘、内分泌失调以及免疫功能低下等病症；可以防治高血压、慢性支气管炎、焦虑症、抑郁症等身心疾病。

Long-term practice of qigong exercise in walking can supplement healthy qi, remove pathogenic qi, eliminate diseases and benefit health. Persistent exercise can regulate Sanjiao, soothe the liver, fortify the spleen and prevent or treat prolapse of internal organs, hypotension, gastrointestinal disorders, constipation, endocrine disorder and immunodeficiency. This exercise can also prevent or treat hypertension, chronic bronchitis, anxiety and depression.

强身健体
Strengthen the Body

　　行步功习练后可以调理身心，祛病健身，日久功深还能增强腿部的功力。通过不断的习练能够开筋通络，增强内气以修成内功，同时锻炼筋骨皮肉，能使我们的身体由弱转强，最后达到内外兼修、强身健体的功用。

The practice of qigong exercise in walking can regulate the body and mind, remove diseases, promote health, and strengthen the legs over time. Through persistent practice, it can strengthen the tendons and unblock meridians, enhance the internal qi to cultivate internal strength, as well as strengthen the muscles and bones. It increases physical strength and benefit health.

行 步 功　● 　*Xing Bu Gong*　(Qigong Exercise in Walking)

The Meridian Charts

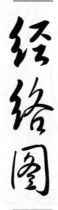

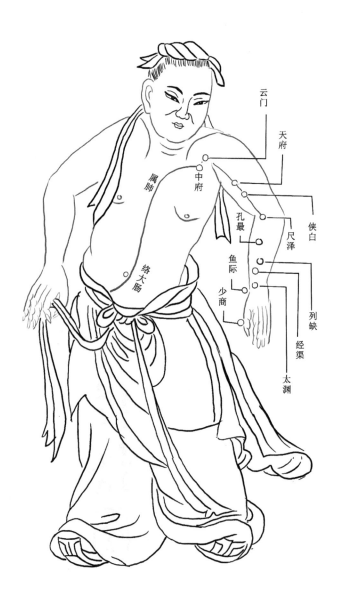

云门

天府

属肺

中府

侠白

孔最

尺泽

鱼际

列缺

少商

经渠

太渊

络大肠

手太阴肺经

Lung Meridian of Hand-Taiyin

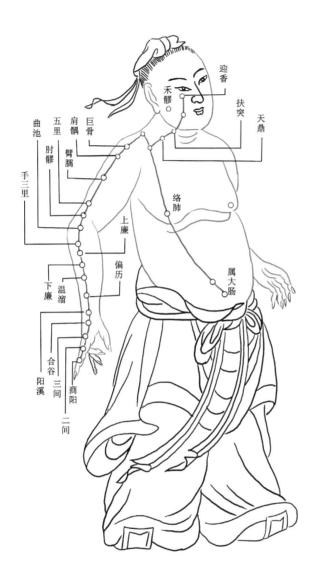

迎香
禾髎
扶突
天鼎
曲池
五里
肩髃
巨骨
肘髎
臂臑
手三里
络肺
上廉
偏历
属大肠
下廉
温溜
合谷
三间
商阳
二间
阳溪

手阳明大肠经

Large Intestine Meridian of Hand-Yangming

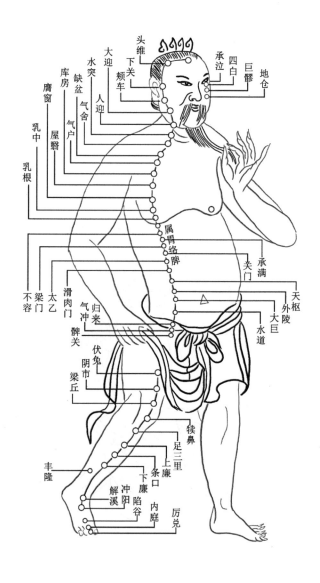

足阳明胃经

Stomach Meridian of Foot-Yangming

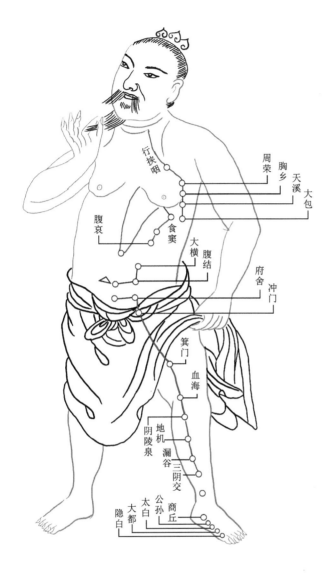

足太阴脾经

Spleen Meridian of Foot-Taiyin

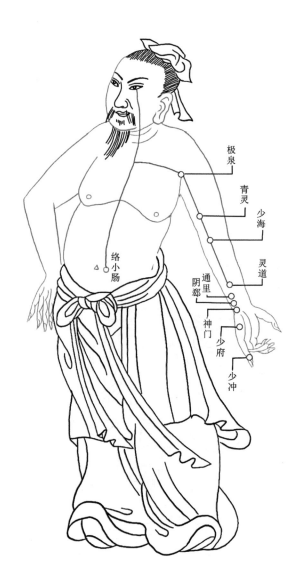

极泉
青灵
少海
灵道
络小肠
通里
阴郄
神门
少府
少冲

手少阴心经

Heart Meridian of Hand-Shaoyin

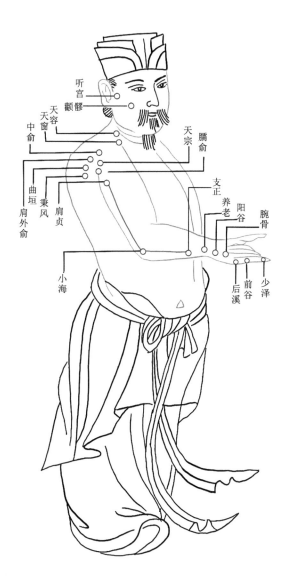

听宫
颧髎
天容
天窗
中俞
曲垣
秉风
肩贞
肩外俞
小海
天宗
臑俞
支正
养老
阳谷
腕骨
后溪
前谷
少泽

手太阳小肠经

Small Intestine Meridian of Hand-Taiyang

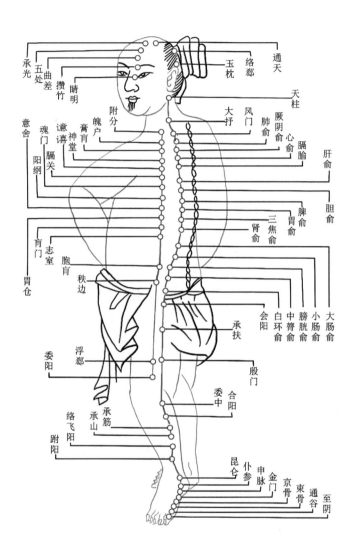

足太阳膀胱经

Bladder Meridian of Foot-Taiyang

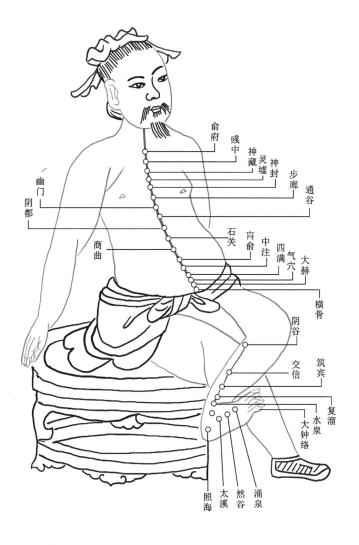

足少阴肾经

Kidney Meridian of Foot-Shaoyin

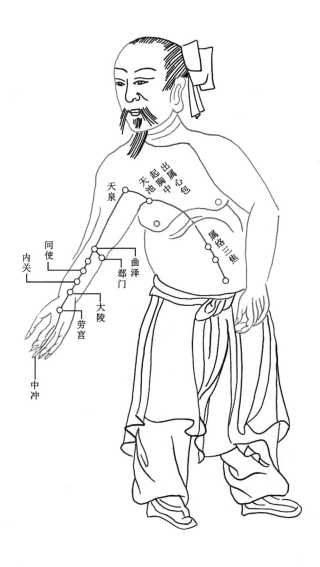

天泉
天池
起胸中
出属心包
属络三焦
间使
内关
曲泽
郄门
大陵
劳宫
中冲

手厥阴心包经

Pericardium Meridian of Hand-Jueyin

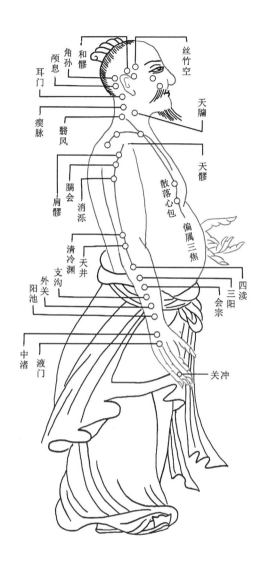

丝竹空
和髎
角孙
颅息
耳门
瘛脉
翳风
天牖
天髎
臑会
肩髎
消泺
散落心包
偏属三焦
清冷渊
天井
支沟
外关
阳池
三阳
四渎
会宗
中渚
液门
关冲

手少阳三焦经

Triple Energizer Meridian of Hand-Shaoyang

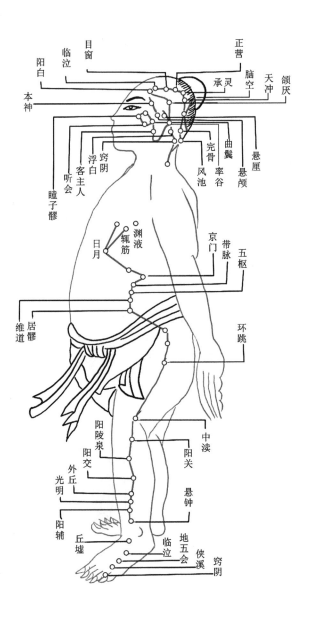

足少阳胆经

Gallbladder Meridian of Foot-Shaoyang

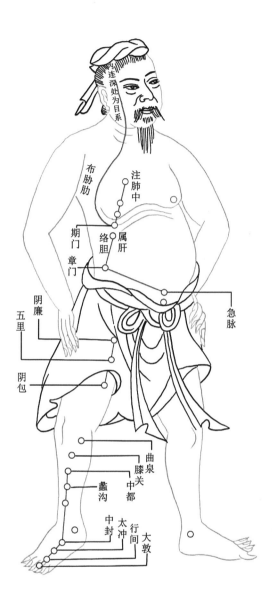

足厥阴肝经

Liver Meridian of Foot-Jueyin

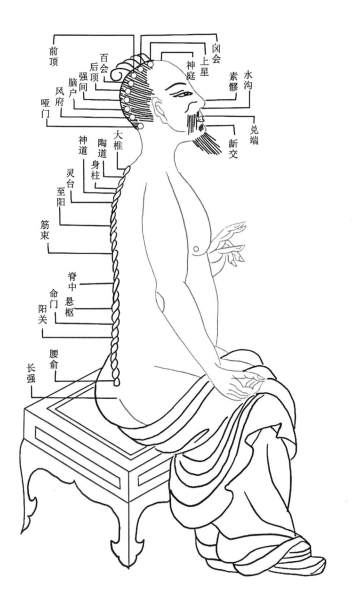

督脉

Governor Vessel (Du)

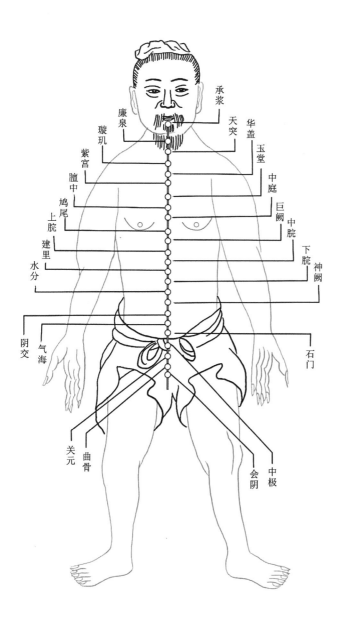

任脉

Conception Vessel (Ren)

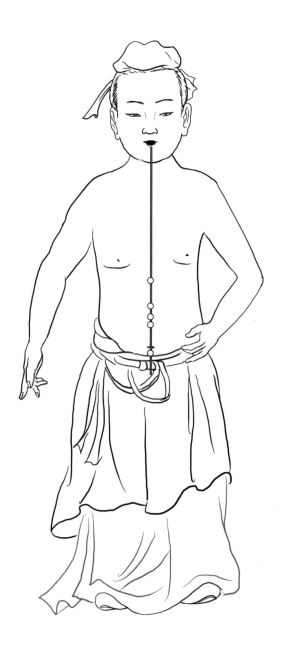

冲脉

Thoroughfare Vessel (Chong)

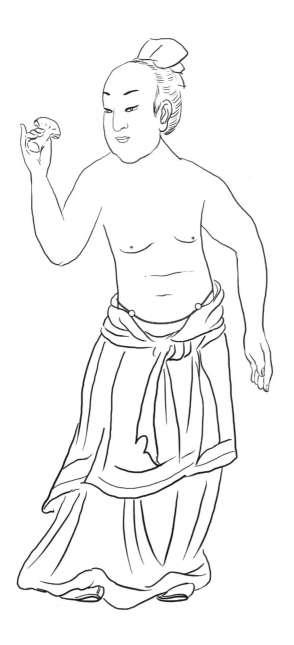

带脉

Belt Vessel (Dai)

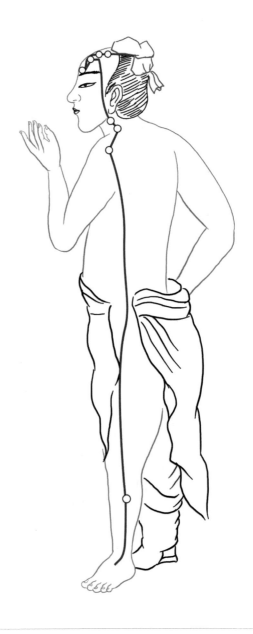

阳维脉

Yang Link Vessel (Yang Wei)

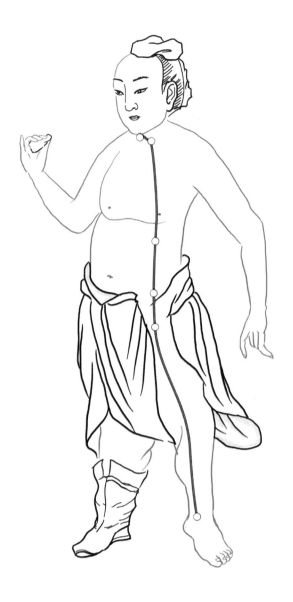

阴维脉

Yin Link Vessel (Yin Wei)

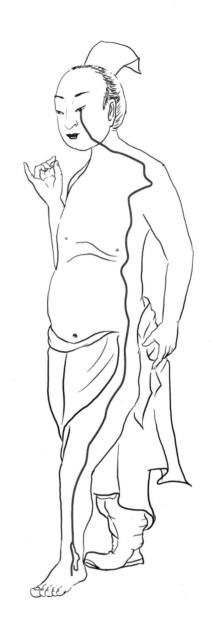

阳蹻脉

Yang Heel Vessel (Yang Qiao)

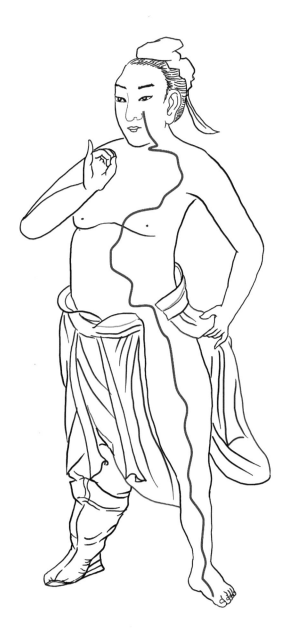

阴蹻脉

Yin Heel Vessel (Yin Qiao)